Where Are the Miracles?

Experiences & testimony of a medical Doctor on the mission field

To Naomi

Best wishes

Dr. Garland Bare

Garland

Lifechange Media
Kearney, NE

LIFECHANGE MEDIA

Library of Congress Cataloging-in-Publication Data

Bare, Garland
Where are the Miracles?
ISBN 978-0-9852128-3-4
1. Christian life. I Title. I. Miracles

First printing: October 2015

Cover design: Lifechange Media
www.Lifechange-Media.com

Printed in the United States by Morris Publishing®
3212 East Highway 30
Kearney, NE 68847
1-800-650-7888

Dedication

This book is dedicated to my tireless companion in writing

Dr. Lynn Gardner

Without whose persistent encouragement the project might never have reached completion.

Contents

With Gratitude for...

My wife, Dorothy and children, Geoffrey, Corrine, and Grace, whose loving contributions and support carried me

Our fellow workers in Thailand who helped to make our ministry possible and encouraged us: Imogene Williams, the C.W. Callaway family, the Byers families, David and Deloris Filbeck, and the De Los Santos family.

Victor Knowles and the Mt. Hope Church of Christ offering a platform to present a preview of this book.

Greg Swinney, David Paine and all the others who gave a boost when I was stalled.

Cindy Swinney, a great encourager who wrote the study questions at the conclusion of each chapter.

All who read the initial manuscripts and gave helpful suggestions: Al & Rhonda Juve, Charlie Shafer, Mike and Robin.

My "Stretcher Bearers" Brian and Ann Lange, Mike Jensen and Jan who carried us through some deep waters.

Foreword

His early religious and scientific training made Garland Bare skeptical about the reality of miracles in today's world. In this book, hc reports experiences in his life and medical ministry that changed his mind. Undeniable evidence led Dr. Bare to believe in miracles occurring today.

The subject of miracles fascinates readers. In February 2015, Amazon.com lists the following numbers of book titles under these topics: miracles—40,351, miracles today—5,977, and healing miracles—19,995. Dr. Bare's eyewitness account provides evidence of the reality of miracles.

Does God still work supernaturally in today's world? Believing that matter is all that exists, atheists cannot have miracles because they have no God to work them. Pantheists believing everything is god cannot have miracles because they believe no personal God exists separate from the world. Everything that exists is god.

For miracles to be a reality, a supernatural God must exist outside the physical universe who can intervene in the physical world. A miracle is an event in the physical world, observable by the senses, worked by the direct power of God. If God created the world and set it up to operate on the basis of what we call natural laws, it would be no problem for Him to adjust nature to operate in a special way for His purpose.

Many assume that believers accept miracles because of their religious dogma and naturalistic scientists reject them because of the evidence. Just the opposite is true. Unbelieving scientists reject miracles because of their worldview dogma of naturalism. In their rejection of miracles, they speak as philosophers, not scientists. Believers accept miracles because of the evidence.

If one grants the possible existence of a supernatural being, then miracles are possible. The key question, "Have miracles occurred in today's world?" must be settled by historical evidence. Do we have credible witnesses that miracles have occurred in the modern world?

To decide the issue of the reality of miracles, we must examine the evidence. We do not have to observe a miracle personally before we can be convinced of the reality of miracles. We did not have to witness the dropping of the atomic bomb on Japan to accept it as a fact. Truth can be communicated by credible eyewitnesses.

In *Where Are the Miracles?* Dr. Garland Bare documents his eyewitness testimony of experiences in his life and medical ministry that he cannot explain by normal, natural processes. He believes they demonstrate the supernatural hand of God. Dr. Bare does not try to force the reader to agree with him. He reports on his experiences in a straightforward, honest way and leaves it for the reader to come to his or her own conclusion.

Dr. Bare tells the story of his first eleven years growing up in Tibet in his earlier book, *A Tibetan Childhood* (Kearney, Nebraska: Lifechange Media, 2012). After high school, he switched from his goal of being an ornithologist and chose to attend Bible college. He decided to be a missionary to the Orient. Since their marriage in 1951, Garland and Dorothy Bare have lived as a team united by faith and dependence upon God, love for God and others, and commitment to God's will regardless of the cost.

The reader will learn the amazing story of how, after serving as a missionary in Thailand, he became a medical doctor and had a medical ministry in Thailand. The reader will ponder these questions: How could a young man with malignant malaria be dramatically healed? How many have enrolled in medical school without funds to pay for tuition yet graduated from medical school debt free? How could a missionary doctor without fundraising end up with an equipped hospital in Pua, Thailand?

Influenced by the example of his parents, as well as the examples of Hudson Taylor and George Mueller, the Bares chose not to use fundraising appeals but prayerfully depended on God for support. While never with an abundance, in remarkable ways their needs were met.

While small in stature, Dr. Bare is strong in spirit, kind, loving, and considerate of others while at the same time determined and methodical in accomplishing what he needs to do. Deeply conscious of his shortcomings he deflects attention from himself by focusing on service to others. This eyewitness narrative provides powerful evidence of the working of God in our world today. Dr. Bare writes his story so that God may be glorified.

H. Lynn Gardner

Reader Testimonials

"The story of what God has done through Dr. Garland Bare is filled with excitement and adventure. You will be inspired to believe with Dr. Bare that God doesn't just open doors. He also knocks down walls. This book by Dr. Bare has inspired me to be a better follower of Christ. I believe it will also do the same for you."

- Boyce Mouton, Minister

"It is a wonderful book. It brought back many memories as well as teaching me many things beyond my child's awareness at the time. I am so glad Dad has written it."

- Corinne Wilson, daughter of Garland & Dorothy Bare

"Along with the medical evidence for miracles presented in the book, the conversion of people like Saeng Pua provides more evidence of a different kind."

- Al Juve, Missionary in Japan

"From one page to another, stories of God's Divine intervention, guidance, protection and provision, fill every chapter of this captivating story. You cannot read this book and remain unchanged. You begin to recount the supernatural work of God in your own life and give thanks for His work in everyone."

- Greg Swinney, International Student Minister

Preface

On the Mekong Trail

The great Mekong River begins as a clear stream fed by snowmelt and springs along the eastern edge of the Tibetan plateau. Rushing through a rift in the Himalayas it roars over boulders beneath towering cliffs. Human conversation becomes impossible on the narrow trails carved out above the foaming rapids. It drops three miles in elevation from the frigid rivulet to the steamy delta at the Gulf of Tonkin.

A sandpiper flying from wintering grounds on a sandbar between Laos and Nan Province in Thailand, en route to its breeding territory in Siberia, would require only 100 miles to reach Tsakalo in Eastern Tibet. The river, with its twists and turns, requires many more miles to cover the same two points on its 2700 mile course from its source in Tibet to the South China Sea.

This book continues the story of the Mekong Trail. It began in my earlier book, *A Tibetan Childhood*, a narrative of my early life on the Tibetan border with my missionary parents.

The story takes up following a decade in the United States where I completed high school and undergraduate college. With my bride Dorothy, in late 1951 we began mission work among the tribes of northern Thailand.

The Mekong River forms the eastern boundary of Thailand. We started more than three decades of observing and learning the surpassing power of a living God, moving above and beyond expectations in the provision of needs, healing of illness, and transforming lives.

The target audience of this testimony is primarily my children and grandchildren, but also all who would explore the greatness of a God who reigns above "natural law." How great is our God!

Introduction

"We have our miracles, but they are all in the Bible," my professor at Abilene Christian College declared. My teachers at the college and College Church in Abilene and later at Lincoln Bible Institute believed the age of miracles ended with the ministry of the apostles. People have always been interested in healing. Do miraculous healings occur today? Or did God only heal miraculously in Bible times?

Dr. William A. Nolen, the author of *The Making of a Surgeon*, observed a strong will to live among his terminal patients. He became interested in the claimed miracles in healing campaigns. After his research, he wrote *Healing: A Doctor in Search of a Miracle* (New York: Random House, 1974). Kathryn Kuhlman, a famous healer of the 1960's and 1970's, held healing campaigns around the country. She had a campaign close to Dr. Nolen's practice in Minneapolis. He volunteered to assist in her campaign, pushing people in wheelchairs and assisting people to the platform. He had the full cooperation of Miss Kuhlman. He believed she was sincere, a well-meaning, basically honest person. With her cooperation and with the permission of some of the patients who had claimed healing in her campaign or had gone forward for healing, he did follow-up studies.

Dr. Nolen found no healings of severed spinal cords, metastatic cancer, congenital brain damage (cerebral palsy), or severe trauma. He did notice that there were at least temporary resolutions of other types of illness. Arthritis improved significantly after the services, whether this was self-hypnosis or actual healing, Dr. Nolen could not determine. People with migraine headaches and other chronic pain syndromes did seem to experience some degree of healing.

He also investigated a man prominent in the 1970's from Houston, Texas, Norbu Chen (Norbu is a Tibetan name and Chen is a Chinese name). This man was an American ex-convict who claimed to have tried to go to Tibet to learn the healing techniques of the Tibetan llamas, but was not permitted. There is a Tibetan kingdom in the Himalayas, independent of China, called Sikkim. Norbu Chen claimed to have gone there receiving instruction and meditation and learning the healing arts of the Tibetans. After investigating his "healings" Nolen concluded he could explain nearly all of them by normal physiological activity rather than miraculous healings.

Also prevalent in the 1970's were the famous Filipino psychic surgeons. Dr. Nolen actually traveled to the Philippines because there were reports from the American Press and even on television of supposed barehanded surgery where these Filipino "surgeons," sometimes with unwashed hands, invaded the abdomen of people and brought up pieces of so-called tissue, which they claimed were appendixes or tumors, leaving the patient without any scars or pain. Dr. Nolan was able to collect some of these specimens and found that they were cotton soaked in a red liquid. He found no real healings by these Filipino psychic "surgeons."

Dr. Nolen concluded, "Two years ago I began looking for a healing miracle. I hoped to find evidence that someone somewhere had supernatural power to cure the 'incurable' . . . I have been unable to find any such miracle worker." I wrote this book in response to this statement.

INTRODUCTION

In my forty-three years of licensed medical practice surprises filled my experience. Patients who seemed on the road to recovery took sudden downturns to unexpected deaths. On the other hand, moribund patients who seemed doomed not to recover have revived and recovered against all the odds. Every year I witnessed remarkable recoveries in response to prayer, but very few that could be scientifically termed miracles.

In this book, I endeavor to narrate accurately some of the events in the lives of my family and my patients that I cannot explain as natural occurrences. The purpose of this book is to tell the facts of these experiences and let you, the reader, decide whether or not they were miracles. Do the experiences reported in this book provide evidence that God continues to work in the world today?

Part One

Medical Experiences of Healing

Chapter 1

Birth Injury

In 1930, my father was the only doctor in the hospital in Batang in Western China. Because of the fighting between Chinese and Tibetans, the border changed back and forth several times, so part of the time Batang was in Tibet and part of the time it was in China. An American missionary nurse, Miss Grace Young, assisted him.

On the date of my birth on a cold January morning, my father was present as my mother was expecting to deliver the baby. Before the birth, he had to leave to attend to a surgical emergency. This left Grace Young to do the delivery. My mother felt that there was something wrong and wondered if the delivery would be breech. Upon my father's return, he was dismayed to find that his newborn son did not have normal muscle tone. He recognized evidence of a brainstem birth injury, which often happens with a breech delivery.

As an infant, my limbs dangled. I could not flex my arms and legs as a normal baby does. My mother worked with me for hours flexing my arms and legs and massaging my limbs. I showed little response, with only gradual improvement. I never crawled, I never learned to roll over, but by the time I was three years old I was beginning to take a few steps, usually with support. I did not have any coordination and fell frequently.

Other evidences of the birth injury included lack of hand-eye coordination. As a boy, I could never catch a football, put a basketball through the hoop, or connect a bat to a baseball. I had a prominent tremor in my hands.

I was three years old when my parents returned for their first furlough to the United States. One of my father's classmates in medical school had become a pediatrician and had a practice in Denver. My parents took me to see Dr. Rex Murphy. He said that no medical treatments existed for what he called hypotonia, but caffeine could be a central nervous system stimulant that might help me. So, at age three I started on my daily cup of coffee, actually it was a cup of milk and sugar with some coffee included in it. Now whether that helped or not, my ability to walk improved and the falls became less frequent. As a small boy, not being able to participate in the games that my brother enjoyed burdened me. While very interested in sports, I always watched from the sidelines.

During high school, I wanted to be a zoologist, particularly ornithology (the study of birds). Most of the science books I could obtain at that time taught Darwinism, and I began questioning my faith under that influence. Finally, I decided that I would go into medicine. I had watched with interest as my father treated his patients in Tibet, but my motives for going into medicine at that time were purely financial. I did not want to live through the poverty and deprivation that my parents had endured in their work among the Tibetans. So I decided that medicine would be my vocation to make money to support my avocation, which would be ornithology.

My senior year in high school in Abilene, Texas, I was president of the premedical club. I had a great deal of difficulty with my uncoordinated hands in the chemistry laboratory. At the end of the school year, Mrs. McCormick, my teacher, called me into her office. She said, "Garland, I know you want to become a doctor, but I've been teaching chemistry for 18 years and I never had a student who spilled so many reagents, messed up so many experiments, or broke so many test tubes as you have. Hold out your hands." I held them out, and they were shaking as usual. She said, "Garland if you were the patient on the table and your life depended on it, would you like hands like that operating on you?"

I said, "No, ma'am." This decided the issue for me. I could never be a doctor. My acceptance of this decision was total. I never grieved or felt regretful over it.

In my subsequent studies of neurology and my work with patients as a physician, I found that most brainstem injuries leave permanent damage to the central nervous system and the musculoskeletal system, so any recovery is generally unexpected. Therapy can improve the performance of available nerve tracts, but there are seldom any direct cures for this. One could rationalize that the improvement allowing me to walk and maintain my sense of balance resulted from therapy and self-effort. However, I did not see that happen in my personal experience with my patients.

During my college years at Lincoln Bible Institute, I experienced weakness in my ankles. I flunked my physical exam, and the military rejected me. They told me I would never be able to do the hiking required by the United States infantry. But, our powerful God, who overcomes what is humanly impossible, accepted me in his service.

I was twenty-one years old when Dorothy and I went to the mission field. I climbed the trails and mountains, being active all the time. We had no motor vehicles in our area, so the choices were walking, horseback riding, or riding a bicycle during the dry season. With no dependence on motor

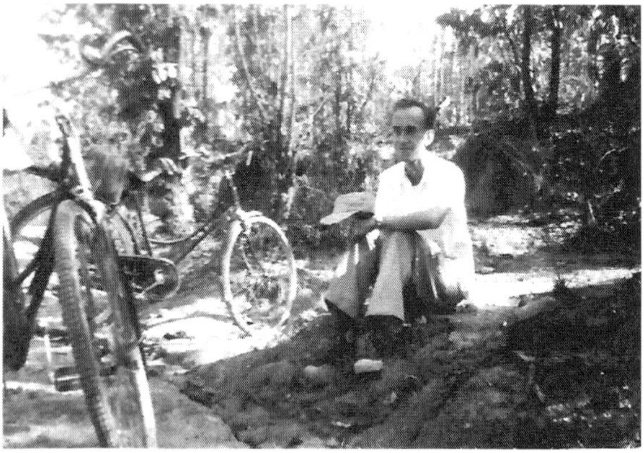

Garland resting during bike ride to remote villages

transportation, I showed continual improvement in strength and in the ability to walk great distances. However, the tremor persisted with my hands.

Years later, in circumstances I will describe later, I was able to go to medical school. By the time I took my premedical courses at Wheaton College, by propping my hands I was able to handle the test tubes and reagents with very little spillage or problems with the experiments required to finish the courses. However, the tremor did persist, making me rather fearful of continuing in medical school. What would happen when I would actually be called to work with living humans, especially in performing surgery?

Walking the trail

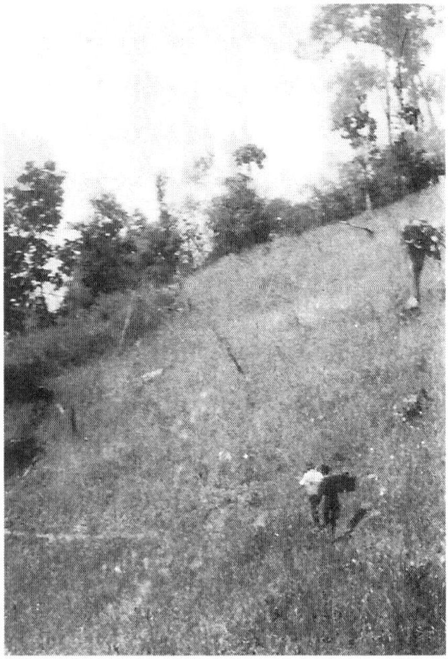

I did manage to be accepted into medical college. During my pre-clinic years, the first and second years of medical school, I was able to do the required science courses--anatomy, physiology, biochemistry, pathology--with minimal clumsiness and spillage. As the time approached when I would be working on human patients, I experienced a combination of fear and assurance that God would somehow get me through this very difficult period.

At the end of my sophomore year in medical school, we had dog labs. Stray dogs were brought in from the street. Students practiced surgery on these dogs including repairing the surgical wounds. We received commendation when the dog survived and recovered. We owned a dog, probably the stupidest dog I've ever known. This extremely fertile dog we called Bugle Ann. I determined that Bugle Ann would never produce any more offspring. I performed a hysterectomy on her for my dog lab project. The operation was a success, and Bugle Ann recovered from the surgery.

In anticipation of working on human subjects, I turned our home into a laboratory. I thank God for the patience of my wife. To learn to do surgical knots, I studied a book on basic surgery and practiced all the surgical knots and sutures. At that time, electrocoagulation was in its infancy, and not available to us. So I got lengths of string and practiced tying surgical knots on the legs of the chairs in our dining room and any other surface. To the exasperation of Dorothy, my wife, I just left the knots in place so when company arrived all these strings were attached to the furniture. Dorothy was rather embarrassed explaining what had happened.

I also read that vascular surgery, which was extremely painstaking, could be practiced by suturing cooked macaroni. The texture of veins is similar to the texture of cooked macaroni. I asked my wife to boil up pots of macaroni and I sutured the elbows end-to-end and practiced it for a long period with little success.

Finally, the day arrived in my junior year of medical school when for the first time I would be assisting surgery on a living patient. I felt an unusual calmness expecting to be terrified, but not experiencing any terror that morning. We had been taught to go through all the steps, the careful scrubbing of the hands and how to cooperate with the operating room nurses when gowned and gloved.

As I scrubbed for surgery that morning, instead of the anxiety I was expecting, I experienced peace and calm in my heart. I walked into the OR, where the nurses were waiting. They gowned me and gloved me, and I walked to the table to assist. My duties were to hold the retractors so the surgeon could see the operating field, to keep the instruments out of the line of his vision, to mop up any pools of blood, and to suture. *My hands did not shake*, and I completed each responsibility. After that, I have never had the tremor. In subsequent years, I have done vascular surgery, brain surgery and operated on every part of the human body. For three years, I served as a war zone surgeon in the war in Southeast Asia.

In 1997, on my first trip back to Abilene since I graduated from high school, I attended and celebrated the fiftieth reunion of my class. I hoped Mrs. McCormick would be present because I wanted to show her my hands and say, "Mrs. McCormick, these are the hands that messed up all the experiments, that spilled all the reagents, that broke all the test tubes. And through the grace and power of God they have done vascular and brain surgery." Unfortunately, Mrs. McCormick had gone to her eternal reward. Classmates who remembered me from fifty years previously expressed surprise at the turn that my pathway in life had taken and were very interested in my missionary experiences.

At age thirty-six, the tremor in my hands that I had experienced since my brainstem birth injury was healed. Not only did the tremor leave my hands, but my eye coordination seemed to be totally healed. I had never been able to play sports before, and now, for the first time in my life, I felt I could participate. When invited, I joined the soccer team in the intramural program at Chiang Mai University. For many years I had watched soccer, the national sport of Thailand. I tried out for the team and made it. The sight of a thirty-six year-old playing with twenty-year-olds amused the crowd. As the only American student among the 6000 students at Chiang Mai University, I was a local curiosity. As we played our game, a roar arose from the crowd every time I would connect with the soccer ball. For the first time in my life, I was a sports celebrity.

During my surgery residency in Omaha a few years later, I exercised in a gym at the medical center. Interns and residents would shoot off steam by going to the basketball court there. Amazingly, when I threw the ball a certain percentage of the time it actually went through the net. Finally, I concluded that I was completely healed of my brainstem injuries.

Study Questions

1. As a small boy, Garland was unable to participate in sports due to his physical limitations and it "burdened" him to watch from the sidelines. Have you had a short-term disability like a broken leg, or a lifelong struggle with a physical limitation? How did you find a way to overcome that feeling of discouragement about being different from others?

2. Read about Jabez in 1 Chronicles 4:9-10. What was his prayer?

3. The Apostle Paul knew the secret to overcoming limitations. Read Philippians 4:13. How are Paul's words similar to Helen Keller's when she said "I thank God for my handicaps for through them I have found myself, my work, and my God."

4. Garland's dream to become a medical doctor was shattered when Mrs. McCormick called attention to his mistakes and shaky hands in the chemistry laboratory. He was later rejected by the military. "But, our powerful God, who overcomes what is humanly impossible, accepted me in his service." Have you had a time or circumstance where you felt God helped you overcome a discouraging time of rejection?

Chapter 2

A Healed Heart

Before we went to the mission field, Dorothy and I had a complete medical check-up and later we had evaluations from the mission hospital in Bangkok. My electrocardiogram had always been normal and my heart was never an issue. During the first term on the mission field, I did suffer a lot of tropical illness, especially after we moved into a primitive area in 1954. I experienced dengue fever, probably malaria, typhoid, amebic dysentery, and numerous tropical parasites. My heart always seemed to be in good shape.

In 1961, David and Deloris Filbeck joined our mission work at Pua. Their oldest son, David, and our son, Geoffrey, shared birthdays a few days apart in March, so we had the birthday party at Filbecks' house. At the party I was leading the children in games when I felt an overwhelming tightness in my chest, accompanied by weakness.

The roads would be opening, and the community of Pua had recently purchased a fire truck. It could come in over the ox cart trail. David Filbeck arranged for the fire truck to take us to our provincial capital at Nan, and there we found a rice truck that was heading over the mountains to Prae, 140 kilometers away where there was a mission hospital. Lying atop the rice truck I felt my strength ebbing. I was getting progressively weaker.

We finally crossed the mountain ranges to Prae. As the truck pulled into the hospital, the truck boys (workers on the truck) unloaded my body from atop the rice truck, and spoke to the man at the emergency room door. I heard them say "The foreigner died on our truck, and it will cost 600 baht [the equivalent of thirty dollars] to exorcise his spirit from the truck." A Thai nurse's aide stepped out of the emergency room door, bent over, and placed her stethoscope on my chest. She said, "I don't hear a heartbeat. He's not moving; he's not breathing."

Then Dr. Steiner, a Mennonite volunteer physician at the hospital, looked out and said, "He's not dead. Get him on oxygen."

During this period, I felt that all my strength was gone. Unable to respond in any way, I could not even open my eyes, but my mind was screaming, "Don't put me in the morgue, I'm still alive!" I prayed, "Lord, I know that Dorothy will be all right, she has strong faith in you, but I have a little boy and a little girl and another one on the way. I'd like to have them grow up with a daddy."

The doctor kept me in the hospital overnight for observation until I could be flown to Chiang Mai the next day. It was quite an experience to be met by the ambulance at the plane door and have the sirens wailing as we rushed to McCormick Hospital. The internist/cardiologist at the hospital took care of me. Meanwhile, Dorothy arrived somehow at the hospital. As I was recovering, the doctors said, "You'll never climb the mountains or walk the trails again, and your life expectancy is not more than five years." My diagnosis proved to be a viral myocarditis. The basic treatment for that is a cardiac transplant, but heart transplants were not done in those days. Without the transplant, there is a very low survival rate.

I decided, rather than taking the advice of the cardiologist, I would commit my case to God and follow the healing advice of Theodore Roosevelt and Dwight D. Eisenhower. The conventional treatment for heart problems was to rest, relax, and wait for the end to come. But Dr. Paul Dudley White, who was Eisenhower's cardiologist at the time President Eisenhower had a heart attack, took the opposite course. He said, "The heart is a muscle and you don't heal muscles by letting them vegetate. The heart has to be rehabilitated like any other muscle." So he put Eisenhower on a vigorous rehabilitation program. This was the beginning of cardiac rehabilitation. I decided that rather than relax and take it easy, I would, as much as possible, rehabilitate my heart by pushing the limit. So I followed Theodore Roosevelt's advice to live vigorously. Instead of resting, I exercised.

After five years were up, Dr. Colbert, the cardiologist at the medical center, said my heart was in good condition. He said the scarring of the heart muscle would always mean abnormal EKG's, but basically my heart was functioning well. When we returned to the United States, I continued my program of living vigorously. When we arrived in Lincoln, Nebraska in 1974 I started a program to climb each of the fifty-nine 14,000 foot peaks in Colorado. I would take a group of students mountain climbing in the summer. I also joined the Century Club. I would run either 100 miles a month or at least 1000 miles in a year. I have felt that my recovery was largely due to divine intervention, but also through cooperation with the best medical help.

Study Questions

1. Have you or a loved one had a near-death experience? What was Garland's prayer when he thought he might die?

2. Read Mark 11:24. Did God answer Garland's prayer with a miracle?

3. Read 1 Peter 5:10. Does God always answer prayers for healing with a miracle? Discuss this statement: "I think God heals everyone who believes; some are healed while they are still here on earth, and the others are healed when they get to heaven."

4. Read Psalm 16. How would this Psalm comfort a person who is facing surgery or even hospice?

Chapter 3

God's Grace for Our Grace

Our daughter, Grace Eileen, was born October 8, 1962 in Thailand. The Thai people could not pronounce Grace, so they called her Eileen, her middle name. To all the Thai people she was Eileen. In the early weeks of her life, we noticed a limpness and weakness on the left side of her body. She experienced normal movement on the right side. By six months, our cheerful little girl was not meeting normal guidelines. At this point, we detected no brain damage.

Being passionate about Bible translation, I worked with the American Bible Society. The existing Thai Bible translation had been translated from the King James Version. In the process, the translation lost the poetic aspects of the biblical text. I participated in translating the Hebrew Old Testament into the Thai language. Both Hebrew and Thai have roots in the Sanskrit language, and both are poetic languages. We finished the Thai Old Testament revision in 1962.

Dr. William Smalley, American Bible Society representative in Thailand, assigned to me a project to write about the plants and animals of the Bible. In the summer of 1963, I needed to submit my final manuscript of *A Translator's Guide to the Plants and Animals in the Bible* to the American Bible Society and begin my pre-medical studies at Wheaton College in Illinois.

Before returning to the United States, we met with a neurologist in Bangkok, who had been trained in New York City by Dr. Greenspan, a foremost pediatric neurologist in the United States. This neurologist helped us set up an appointment with Dr. Greenspan so he could examine our daughter.

We confronted a serious challenge to our scheduled trip to the United States in 1963. For more than a year, I had experienced attacks of excruciating flank pain. Since I was unable to pass the kidney stones, doctors determined I needed surgery. It could make me miss my scheduled appointments in Israel, London, New York, and Wheaton. Theo Ziemer, a praying missionary, told Dorothy, "There is going to be no surgery."

The morning for the surgery arrived. They prepped me for surgery. While they were wheeling me to the operating room, I passed the stones. Crisis avoided!

Ruth Hardy, a Christian Missionary and Alliance missionary, later asked us if anything had happened on a specific date. She said she had a strong urge to pray for Garland Bare. She went into her bedroom and prayed for me at the exact time I passed the stones.

On the way to the United States, I managed to complete some projects on the Old Testament translation into Thai and research dealing with the plants and animals of the Bible. Our journey back to the states led us first to Jordan and then to Jerusalem. I checked to see if the Dead Sea Scrolls had any useful plant or animal references.

The Hebrew University, on the Jewish side of Jerusalem, was not controlled by Jordan at the time. Before our visit I had contacted Dr. Aharon Shulov, the head zoologist at the university. Dr. Shulov had started the biblical zoo near

Jerusalem, in which he had tried to collect a specimen of every species of animal and bird mentioned in the Bible. He helped me with the identification of animals in the Bible.

Not only did he help in that aspect, but he found out that my wife and children were sitting in a hotel in Jerusalem. He gave up his Sabbath to take us on a tour of Jerusalem and the surrounding area. He took us to his home in the kibbutzim, a communal settlement, so we got to see life in the kibbutzim.

From Jerusalem, we went to Tel Aviv to meet the foremost botanist who helped me with the plant life of the Bible. I discovered that the word *Gilgal* in Hebrew meant anything that rolled across the country, such as a wheel or a whirlwind. My contribution to the New International Version of the Bible was the word *tumbleweed* found twice in the Old Testament (Psalm 83:13; Isaiah 17:13). We went to London to the Kew Botanical Gardens in Kensington, and I observed specimens of actual plant life like those in ancient Israel in Bible times.

Proceeding on our journey, we flew to New York City. After landing at Idlewild (now JFK) Airport, we planned to go to a mission hostel on Long Island where returning missionaries could stay for a nominal fee. Our western clothes were five years out of date. We planned to buy clothes and update our wardrobe. My wife and I did not want to look "mishy" when we presented ourselves to the churches.

In the airport, when I arrived at the baggage claim, a page announced on the loud speaker system, "Mr. Bare, Mr. Garland Bare, please pick up the nearest white phone." I picked up the phone, and a representative of the American Bible Society said he had arranged for someone to pick us up and take us to a suite in the Park Plaza Hotel close to the American Bible Society headquarters, where I could complete my work on the plants and animals of the Bible. Here we were, in our shabby clothes and battered old suitcases, walking through the lobby of this posh hotel. We looked at the expensive food prices in the hotel and nearby restaurants. We ended up getting apples, crackers, and milk and eating in our room.

In the next few days, I finalized the manuscript for my book, *A Translator's Guide to Plants and Animals in the Bible* (American Bible Society, 1963).

We kept our appointment with Dr. Greenspan at his office located near our hotel. We were anxious about what he might charge. We had limited financial resources. We had not purchased anything on credit and did not have a credit card. We found Dr. Greenspan to be a genuine and helpful person.

He examined our eight-month-old daughter, Grace Eileen. After he had examined Grace, he said, "I don't have good news for you. She has cerebral palsy, due to a birth injury, with profound mental retardation. She will never walk properly. She will never talk and will not relate to you normally. My advice is that you do not take her back with you when you go to Thailand because she will be a full-time care project and would interfere with your medical studies and medical practice. She means a lot to you because she is your daughter; you mean nothing to her."

Dr. Greenspan continued, "Now my normal fee is [he mentioned a rather exorbitant amount, more than we had]. I am a Hebrew; I am not a Christian. But I believe in what you are doing, and for you there is no charge for my services." Earlier he had asked about our plans and I told him of my plan to complete pre-med in the United States and go back to Thailand to be a medical student in preparation for a medical mission.

At that time CT scans and MRI's had not yet been developed; the technology did not provide a way of looking inside Grace's brain to see what was really going on. Years later in the 1980s, an MRI showed that Grace had only one hemisphere in her brain. The second hemisphere was only rudimentary. This condition is known as the Dyck-Davidoff-Masson Syndrome. In the 1980s when we learned her condition, recorded medical history knew of only sixty people with this syndrome and none had developed mentally. Most cases never walked or talked and died fairly early.

In spite of Dr. Greenspan's advice, we took Grace with us back to Thailand. She was our daughter, and we were not going to leave her in a United States institution while we returned to Thailand.

In my medical studies in Chiang Mai, the medical center had a brand new physical therapy department, which included speech therapy. The service cost me nothing as a student there. The enthusiastic young therapists spent lots time with Grace. By the time she was two years old she was speaking in sentences in three languages, and by the time she was three she was walking with braces

While I was still in medical school, a Canadian neurologist, Dr. Steele, came out to give lectures at the medical center, and he agreed to evaluate Grace Eileen. He said that definitely some areas in the brain were not functioning normally, but he would expect her to be able to graduate from the eighth grade. In succeeding years, she graduated from high school and took classes at the University of Nebraska until she decided to go to Texas with her boyfriend and get married. They had a beautiful son who is mentally and physically a superb specimen. Her husband was later institutionalized for mental illness. As a paranoid schizophrenic, he was a danger to Grace and their son. At present he lives in a half-way house under supervision. My wife and I became his guardians.

In 2008, when we moved to Spring River Christian Village in Joplin, Missouri, Grace was permitted to live in the assisted living area. She reads to blind residents and serves as an errand girl for our activities director. God has granted his grace to our Grace. By God's grace, our Grace is happy and enjoys worshiping with fellow believers at the Village.

Study Questions

1. A "praying missionary" told Dorothy that there would be no surgery despite firm plans in place for Garland's kidney stones to be removed. A second missionary had felt a strong urge to pray for Garland at a particular time for an unknown reason. Can you think of someone you would consider a prayer warrior for others? Does God hear the prayers of missionaries and ministers more than He hears the prayers of ordinary people?

2. Are there prayers that God does not hear? Read John 9:31, Psalm 66:16-20, and Isaiah 59:2

3. Doctors examined Grace Eileen and said she had profound mental retardation along with other serious physical problems. Institutional life was the best option

for her future, yet Garland and Dorothy took Grace back to Thailand. By age two she spoke three languages, and went on to take college classes and serve God in amazing ways throughout her adult life. Grace still lives with cerebral palsy, so do you think there was a miracle somewhere in her story?

Chapter 4

A Healing from Malignant Malaria

I have experienced God's power and partnership in my medical practice in many ways. I have seen many patients, who were not expected to live, recover against all odds. Yet the recovery could still be explained in physiological terms. So it would be hard to term these recoveries as miracles, but certainly they were above and beyond what would be expected. I believe in the power of prayer. Studies have indicated that faithful and focuesed prayer has healing power.

In forty-three years of medical practice, remarkably few cases could be determined to be miraculous because they transcended the expected physiological pathways of healing. I would like to share with you one such case, a remarkable case, of Banchong, a young man nineteen years old. He was a member of the Blue Hmong tribe. His father was a witch doctor, but his uncle had become a zealous Christian. A cousin witnessed to Banchong and encouraged him to become a Christian.

His witch doctor father found out Banchong was becoming interested in Christianity. He sent him up into the mountains, miles away from the village, to isolate him from the influence of Christians and where hopefully he would get over his desire to follow Christ. The winter of 1972 was particularly disastrous in that it did not get cold enough to kill the *anopheles* mosquito, which is the carrier of malaria, so an ongoing malarial epidemic persisted all that fall and winter. Many people came down with it, overloading our little hospital with patients.

Banchong's family brought him down to the hospital in extremely critical condition. Banchong's blood test showed that he had falciparum malaria. A disease resistant to most of the modern anti-malarial medications we had, including Fansidar, the most effective and safest anti-malarial agent at that time. For forty-eight hours, we tried every medical treatment available, but to no avail. His condition worsened.

We did not have a blood bank because we only had twelve hours of electricity in our hospital each day. So we had to find a donor and the only donor we could find to cross-match with Banchong was a ninety-pound cousin, who had volunteered to donate a unit of blood. But that blood was not effective.

In extreme cases like this, the only solution was to do an intravenous quinine drip. Quinine, the original medication used on malaria, can have highly toxic affects. There is a condition among the peoples of Asia known as G6PD deficiency, which causes abnormal responses to some medications, including abnormal bleeding. People with this deficiency, if they use quinine, will often hemorrhage and pass large quantities of dark blood, a condition known as blackwater fever. It is almost always fatal.

Banchong's father, the witch doctor, came to me and said, "Can God heal my son?'"

I responded, "God can do all things."

"If Banchong becomes a Christian, will he be healed?"

I said, "There is no guarantee that he will be physically healed. He will be spiritually healed if he comes to Christ."

The father urged, “Well, pray for my son that he will be healed.” Banchong was slipping in and out of consciousness; his eyes were becoming glazed, and his extremities were cold. I asked the nurse on duty, who was a committed Buddhist and rather anti-Christian in her outlook, to do vital signs on Banchong. She reported, "The blood pressure is fifty over zero. His pulse is weak, and his respirations are irregular."

"One year ago I forbade my son to become a Christian, but now I am willing if he wants to," the father said.

I asked, “Banchong, last year you were talking about coming to Christ. How do you feel about it now?”

“Doctor, it’s too late.”

“Why is it too late?”

“Because I’m dying, I cannot be baptized. If it is at all possible, I want to be saved.”

I said, “Would you be willing to commit whatever life you have into God’s hands?”

Frustrated, he said, “I can’t pray because of the spirit strings tied around my ankles and wrists.” Spirit strings are associated with demon worship.

So I went to the nurse’s desk, got the scissors, and cut the strings around his ankles and wrists. Then I said, “Now, tell God what you would like to tell Him.”

He prayed, “God, I’ve wanted to follow you for a year and now I am relying entirely on your mercy because I cannot obey you in any way.” Immediately, his eyes brightened up; his color turned to normal, and his extremities started warming. The biggest miracle, the biggest event that I cannot explain, is that the accumulated blood that had puffed up his abdomen disappeared, and it was not passed in any normal way.

I asked the nurse to come back to take Banchong's vital signs. She responded that his blood pressure was approximately 110 over 70; his pulse was about 80 per minute and regular, and his respirations were normal. Banchong's recovery occurred on a Friday. I kept him overnight for observation. The hospital dismissed him on Saturday, a recovering man.

As the members of the refugee church, to which Banchong's uncle belonged, assembled for Sunday morning services, Banchong walked into the assembly to a huge round of applause. All the family and church members had expected a funeral to take place. Banchong confessed his faith in Christ. The entire congregation walked with him a quarter mile to the lake where he was baptized into Christ and began a new life, spiritually and physically. His family was baptized later.

This is one dramatic case for which I could find no medical explanation. You, the reader, will have to decide whether it was a miracle or not. Twenty-three years later I returned to Thailand and found Banchong to be a sturdy, middle-aged elder of the church and in excellent health.

Study Questions

1. Banchong's story was one that Garland described as "a remarkable case." His health was rapidly deteriorating when his father, the witch doctor, said, "Can God heal my son?" What was Garland's response?
2. Banchong's father had a question that is still asked frequently today. Can becoming a Christian heal me? We might hear something like this: "If I accept Jesus as

my Lord and Savior, will my life suddenly become perfect?" How did Garland answer this question?

3. Read James 5:14-16. Most churches no longer anoint the sick, but prayers of faith in difficult situations are commonplace. According to verse 16, what two things are we to do when we desire healing from God?

4. Read Psalm 30. David wrote this psalm, and he had his share of tearful nights and joyful mornings. King Saul tried to kill him, then was killed himself in battle and David occupied the throne as King. David wept when his adultery with Bathsheba was hidden, but experienced joyful mornings once he confessed his sin to God. Banchong survived his "weeping night" of malaria, and a "joyful morning" arrived. What happened after Banchong was healed physically?

Part Two

Provision for Ministry

Chapter 5

Dependence upon God for Support

I would like to make a disclaimer. The Lord gives us tremendous freedom in our method of evangelism. The message remains the same; the method (including how one chooses to be supported) can change.

The Word of God dictates our message and we should not stray from that. We must be absolutely certain what the Bible teaches about the plan of salvation before we try to reach out and teach others the plan of salvation. We are bound by the Word of God and His commandments, so we do not have the latitude to stray from biblical teaching and commands.

On the other hand, the methods for carrying forth that message are limited only by the imagination of man. The early disciples who were with Jesus walked with the Good News wherever He led. Now we can transport the Good News by a variety of means. Distances that covered weeks and months can now be covered in hours. The instruments used for teaching have greatly expanded in our electronic age. We have radio, television, video, the internet, cell phones, and many ways of communicating the Gospel. God has blessed all of these methods with souls won to Christ.

Christians use many options for support for going out as missionaries with the Word: a cooperative group, a mission board, going out as individuals, supported by local churches. In some countries with restrictions on evangelism, missionaries go as tentmakers, carrying their skills and occupations and sharing the gospel in a more limited, yet effective way.

What about support? The Bible does encourage faith and trust in God. After years of observing various methods of missionary support, I believe that as long as missionaries are true to the message of the Word and the plan of salvation, God blesses the means of support equally. Looking at missionaries who raised their support before going out to the field, and those who chose not to, I can see no significant difference. Those who choose to raise support are in no way inferior or superior to those who go out without fundraising.

My parents left the Disciples of Christ mission board in 1933. The Disciples used the economic depression as an excuse for closing down the Tibetan work. My parents determined to go back because they felt that God's call for them had not ended at that time. They had been influenced by their friends of the China Inland Mission, started by Hudson Taylor, in never making financial appeals to raise their support. So my parents returned to the field in the middle of the Depression with four children and no fundraising.

When Dorothy and I decided to go out to Thailand in Southeast Asia, we considered various methods. Some leaders of Lincoln Bible Institute advised us to send out a fund-raising letter to raise funds to cover our expected expenses there. However, we had both been so influenced by the life of Hudson Taylor and George Mueller in trusting God for finances that there were some misgivings when we sent out our fundraising letter. After paying the costs of a newsletter and mailing involved in this, we experienced a net loss of $15.00. We examined our stance and decided never again would we ask people for money. Even though we made this decision we respect those who use fundraising and support those who use this method.

It embarrasses me when people praise me for going out without fundraising. It was because of the weakness of my faith that I chose not to depend on pledged support or on any organization. I remembered the statement in the hymn "Stand Up, Stand Up for Jesus," "The arm of flesh will fail you. You dare not trust your own." Hudson Taylor said he chose to be shipwrecked on God rather than having any other source upon which to depend. I needed to be in a situation where I would put my trust entirely in God.

We would try to raise up an army of prayer supporters. We tried to recruit two hundred people to pray that God would provide our needs. In the following twenty-three years of trusting that God would supply our needs, we saw the bank account hit zero again and again. But there was always a roof over our heads, food on the table, adequate clothing, and in remarkable ways, our needs were met for our work on the mission field. We were able to build a house and a hospital with equipment and staff.

Dorothy agreed to go as a missionary with me to Tibet. I already knew the language, the culture, and the people. We could not go to Tibet because the Chinese Communist takeover of Tibet made it a closed field to missionaries.

My mother told me the C. W. Callaways impressed her. They had attended Cincinnati Bible Seminary. They went initially as missionaries to Burma but had to leave when it became socialist. They did language study in China. Lora Banks, one of the China missionaries, came back to the United States and married Willis Harrison, and C.W. and Lois Callaway and Imogene Williams went to Thailand.

I wrote to C. W. Callaway saying we were considering Thailand as an alternate mission field since we could not go to Tibet. I explained that I only had a bachelor's degree and a year of ministry. I said I needed some graduate work and more ministry experience. He wrote back, "We need you now. We may have only two years. You already know the Yunnanese language (a form of Mandarin Chinese) and will be able to communicate with the people."

We spent our initial two years in Thailand with the C.W. Callaway family. They prepared meals and we studied the language. Then we had to decide where would be the best place to start our outreach with the tribespeople. We had been very

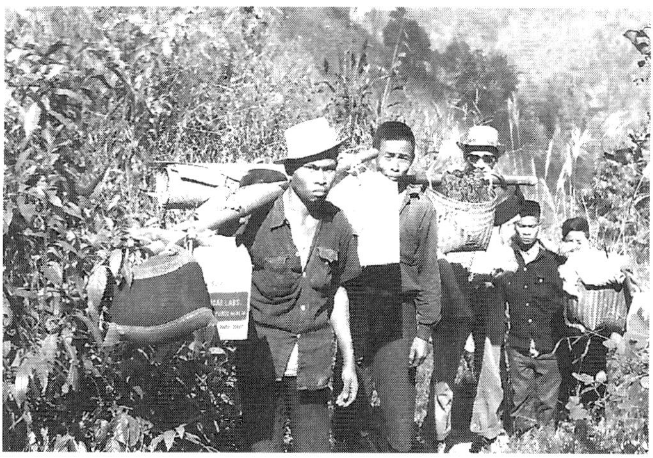

Porters from Lu Tribe with C.W. Callaway (dark glasses)

much attracted to the Blue Hmong tribe. Mr. Callaway and I went on trips surveying areas as possible locations for reaching this particular tribe. First, we went up to Chiang Khong on the Mekong River bordering Laos. Then we made a trip down to Nan Province, where we surveyed the Pua district.

Then we reported back to the missionary group in Chiangkham, which consisted of the Callaways, Dorothy Uhlig, and Imogene Williams. We prayed about the matter as to where we should go following the completion of our language study in Chiangkham. I felt strongly attracted to the northern area around Chiang Khong, but the majority of the missionaries felt that it would be best to settle and work in Nan Province.

In 1954, we moved down to Pua. Quite an adventure, because our possessions went by ox cart and truck to Lampang and on to Nan. Then we had a four-day trip up to Pua, partly by riverboat and partly with an ox cart, while we walked. Our possessions included an ox cart full of commentaries, lexicons, Bible study resources--necessities for translation and conversation work. Everything on that ox cart could now be contained on a computer.

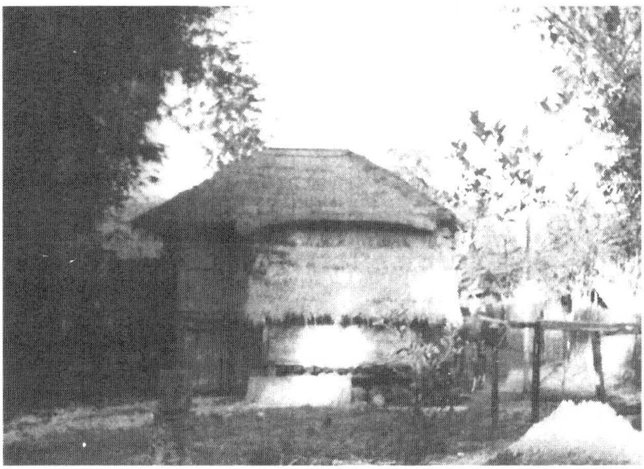

First house in Pua

We went into Pua, a community cold and unfriendly to outsiders. The district had never had any American residents, and the people were quite suspicious of us. Being accustomed to the friendliness of the people around Chiangkham, we felt more or less rebuffed in Pua. We looked around for a place to live and located an available house on the edge of town, which was in great need of repair. In fact, it was like most Thai homes, built up on poles, but the house leaned so badly that we could not move our things into it. So we hired an elephant for $5.00 to pull the house upright. We filled in dirt around the posts before we could move our possessions into the house.

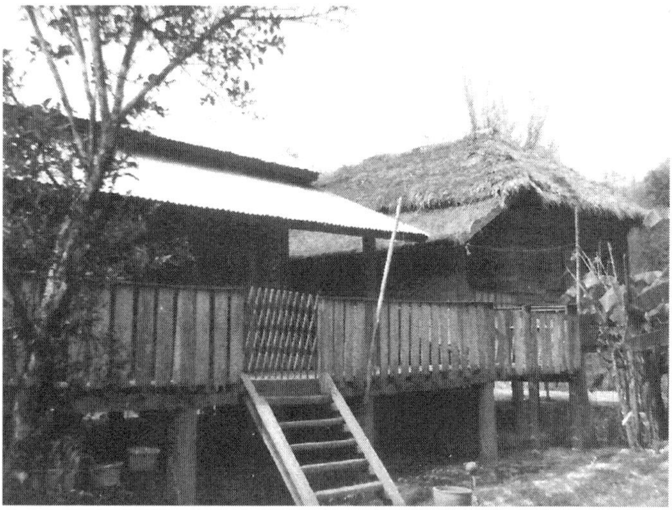

Second house in Pua, also a guest house and hostel for Hmong students

The community had no sewage or sanitation, no electricity, and we started under a leaky roof. One of the first things, after we had pulled the house upright and moved our belongings into it, was to put up a fiberboard ceiling, which we got from the Danish forestry people in Prae. We thought it was a good idea to have a ceiling between us and the leaky roof. The roof was repaired and the ceiling installed. Unfortunately, the ceiling became a race course for rats, and at night while we were trying to sleep, the rats ran back and forth on the loud fiber board. It was quite a disturbance.

My wife, Dorothy was not fond of cats, but when the choice came to cats or rats, she broke down and we got a cat to reduce the rat population. There was quite a bit of curiosity as to our motive for being there in Pua. Very slowly we began to make friends of the community.

Mel Byers came down from Chiangkham to Northern Thailand, and we went on a survey trip to the villages of the Blue Hmong tribe. We called an area on the border of Laos the "frost pocket" because as far as we knew it was the only area in Thailand where it got cold enough to have a frost and occasional ice on the stream. A very influential man in the large village of Kang Haw welcomed us warmly. We were able to communicate because he also spoke the northern Thai dialect.

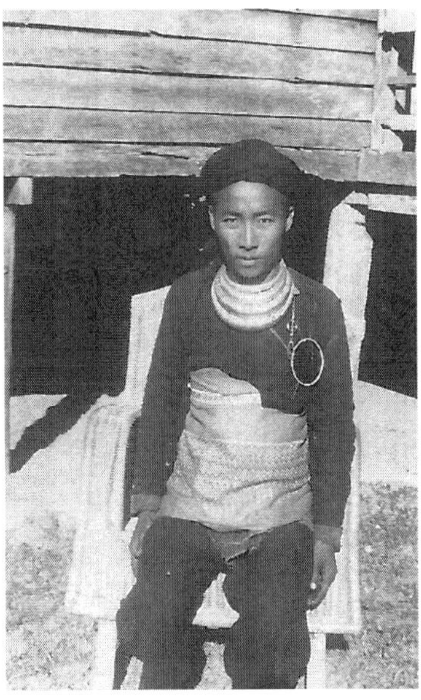

Hmong tribesman in our first home in Pua (1954)

He was extremely curious as to why we would come so far from our homes.

We explained to him that when the sun went down in Thailand it rose up in America and vice-versa. This astounded him. He asked, "Why would you leave your parents and family to come way over here?"

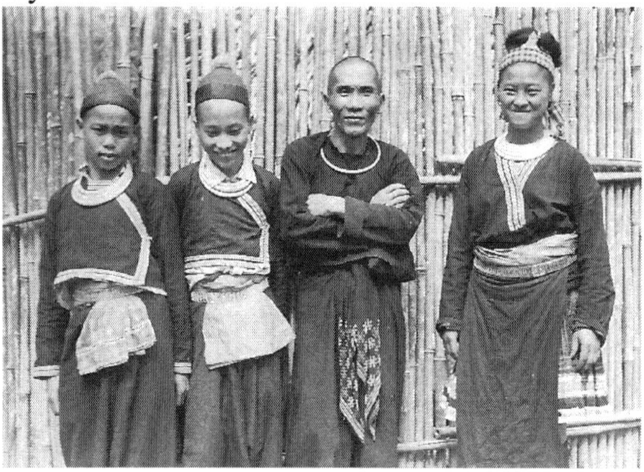

Hmong family outside our bamboo fence

So we accordingly explained that our purpose was to bring the good news of Jesus, who has power over the evil spirits that enslave the animistic Hmong tribe. He questioned us far into the night and was genuinely impressed by the gospel message. He said, "This message must be really important if you would come so far to bring it to us. When you come back and teach us more, we may be ready to believe." Regrettably, the chieftain died before we could make a return trip to the village.

Study Questions

1. It might look as though Garland and Dorothy took a huge step of faith when they decided not to ask people to provide money for their mission work in Thailand. But when praised for going out without fundraising, Garland said there was a different reason for not depending on pledged support. What was it? How does that make sense?

2. Rather than raising money, for what did the Bares ask?

3. Prayer is not merely getting our needs met. It is a culture of dependence. It is a lifestyle of trust and total obedience to God's will and purpose. Is it *easier* to depend on another person to meet your needs, or to depend entirely on God? Why?

4. Read Philippians 4:6. In what situations should we pray?

5. When the Bares found only a rundown house for their family, the Pua community watched curiously trying to determine their motive for being there. When asked "Why would you leave your parents and family to come way over here?" what was Garland's answer?

6. Read Matthew 28:19-20. What command did Jesus give? What promise did he leave us?

Chapter 6

Provision for Our Housewarming

After settling in Pua, we made frequent trips up to the tribal villages. We shared the gospel message charts and recordings that had been produced by the Far East Broadcasting Company in Manila. It is customary among the tribes that if you stay in anyone's home, you invite them to stay in your home. Well, there were hundreds of the tribespeople and only one of our family in Pua. The tribespeople accepted the invitation to our home, and it became very crowded at night. They appreciated being in a place where they felt loved and welcomed rather than with the Chinese merchants in Pua who obviously despised them.

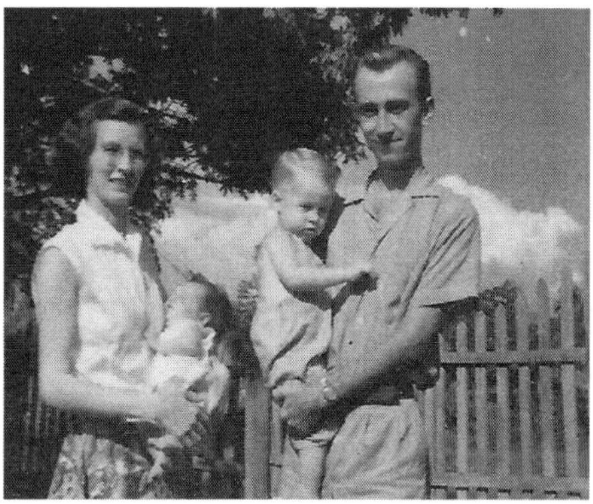

Garland, Dorothy, Geoffrey and Corinne (1956)

PROVISION FOR OUR HOUSEWARMING

In our first three years of marriage, Dorothy experienced two miscarriages. On our next trip to Bangkok, we did a fertility consult at the mission hospital. The doctors evaluating her said that because of fibroid tumors on the uterus Dorothy would not likely be able to carry a pregnancy to term.

On our return trip from Bangkok, we stayed in the guest house of Overseas Missionary Fellowship. The Heimbachs, who managed the guest house, had a four-year-old boy named Danny. Missionary children customarily addressed other adult missionaries as *uncle* and *auntie*. Little Danny climbed onto Dorothy's lap and said, "Auntie, do you have a little boy?"

Dorothy said, "No. I don't have a little boy."

"Would you like to have a little boy?" Danny inquired.

"I would love to have a little boy."

He said, "Well if we ask Jesus, He can give you a little boy." So the little four-year-old prayed, "Dear Jesus, please give Auntie a little boy." He got down off of her lap, and before going to play, turned and said, "Auntie, next year you are going to have a little boy."

Meanwhile, a missionary doctor, Dr. Clarence Yand was visiting and he had been doing research at the University of Washington School of Medicine. He found in cases of miscarriage with women with fibroid tumors that taking thyroid pills helped to take a pregnancy to full term. So he placed Dorothy on thyroid medication and the next year (1955) our little boy, Geoffrey was born. His sister, Corinne, came along the following year.

New recruits came out to help us, so we were able to rent and move to a better house. Don and Roberta Byers joined us in the work in Pua and stayed in the initial home. The tribespeople continued to come in large numbers. When our son, Geoffrey, was born, the people were fascinated by their first view of a white baby. The tribespeople were not noted for their personal hygiene. The people who came evidenced active cases of tuberculosis and even leprosy. We felt very uncomfortable in seeing these diseased and dirty people holding our baby. So we decided to turn our second home into a hostel where the tribespeople could stay at night. We built ourselves a home in the back yard, where we could keep our children safe.

The Byers family planned to start working with the Khamu tribe, so after their basic language study in Pua, they moved to Yao River Valley, where they built a home and worked among the Khamu. This work with the Khamu continued when they moved to California later along with many Khamu refugees.

After a few years, the David Filbeck family came to join us there. Before the Filbecks arrived, we decided to build our "dream house" in the backyard of our current house. The house was pretty much Thai style except we were going to have two innovations--indoor plumbing and screened windows, meaning no longer sleeping under mosquito netting. A young Christian carpenter volunteered to come help us build a new house in exchange for room and board. He was very careful in selecting termite-proof lumber, including teak wood and Thai redwood because the termites were ever present.

It was customary when a house was completed to give a house-warming feast for the village. But when the building was completed, and the carpenters paid off, we found our finances inadequate for an acceptable feast. We recalled that there was a Chinese merchant on the river port, sixteen kilometers away from us. He had asked us to write him a check so that when he went to get merchandise in Bangkok he would not have to take cash. There had been some robberies on the road to Bangkok, so he wanted to avoid that. Trusting there would be money in the bank by the time he went to Bangkok, I wrote him a note asking if we could give him a check for 1500 baht ($75.00 U.S.) in order for us to provide a feast for the villagers. Our carpenter, Jamlong, was to ride his bicycle the next day with the letter and check to see if he could bring back the cash.

At breakfast the next morning, before Jamlong, the carpenter, went down for the money, I had written a letter for him to take to the merchant. To our surprise, the merchant showed up at breakfast time, splattered with mud because it was the rainy season. He said, "Do you people need 1500 baht?"

I said, "Yes, we do. I have a letter here that I wrote to you asking if you could advance it and take our check to Bangkok."

He said, "Well, last night I dreamed that you needed 1500 baht. I felt foolish, but I brought the money." I showed him the letter.

He said, "My, you serve a powerful God."

We were able to buy a hog, have it butchered, and buy enough rice and hot peppers to make a feast for the four hundred guests that came for the housewarming. The guests were impressed with the screened windows, but especially the indoor plumbing. We overheard some of them say, "Why would anyone want to go potty inside their house?" This is one of the many instances where God intervened financially in a seemingly impossible situation. This event helped us establish ties with the community.

We are thankful that as our children were growing up they had the company of the Byers children who were in the same age group, and later the arrival of the Filbecks, so that our children did not grow up entirely without the company of fellow American children. Our children became fluent in the local Thai dialect and also picked up some tribal words and phrases. It has been a joy to see not only our own children, but the Byers and Filbeck children continue in the service of the Lord.

Study Questions

1. Infertility is a heartbreaking problem for couples, and the Bares were no different. But the sincere prayer of a 4-year-old boy was powerful enough to overcome the odds of remaining childless. Read Luke 18:16-17. Characteristics of children include innocence, openness, trust, amazement, wonder, receptivity, confidence, humility. Adults often display skepticism, mistrust, and self-reliance. With all the trials of daily life, can adults really go back to having a childlike faith?
2. When a doctor says "no children" yet the woman becomes pregnant, is that just getting lucky ….. or is that a miracle?
3. Has there been a time when money has unexpectedly arrived at just the right time to meet your financial needs?

4. Garland shared the housewarming story of God's financial intervention in a seemingly impossible situation. The feast met their monetary needs for the food, and also helped establish ties with the community. Does God really know and care about our monthly bills and financial struggles?

5. Read Matthew 6:25-34. Which of our needs does Jesus tell us to worry about?

6. What would your life look like if you were truly seeking God's kingdom and His righteousness?

Chapter 7

Admission to Medical School

1962 was a pivotal and traumatic year in our missionary career. The myocarditis (heart muscle infection) that nearly cost my life was a turning point. Having been informed that my life expectancy was less than five years, how should I plan for the future? Most of the revision of the Thai Old Testament had been completed. I was still working on a translator's guide to the plants and animals of the Bible. Visits to Israel and London would complete the project. I also wanted to help finish a new translation of the New Testament for the Hmong people.

We returned from Chiang Mai to Pua for recuperation and consideration of our future. As usual we had a large number of visitors on a daily basis, including two young Peace Corps volunteers, Brady Deaton and Fred Perry. In later years, we found that both men went on to distinguished careers in the fields of public service and education. At this writing, Dr. Brady Deaton has retired as Chancellor of the University of Missouri.

While hospitalized for the cardiac problems, I had invited Dr. James Steiner of Prae and Dr. Edwin McDaniel of McCormick Hospital to visit Pua and help out on some of the more difficult cases we had tried to treat. Because our district had no trained medical personnel, sick people swarmed to our door. The strong tradition of medical missions in Thailand led to the erroneous belief that all American missionaries were trained healers. Since my father and younger sister were both physicians, they had loaded us with medical books.

For many years we had been praying that God would send us a doctor to free me for Bible translation and evangelism. We had voiced our need for a doctor in our prayer letters. Two American doctors who contacted us backed off when they found out there were no all-weather roads or dependable sources of electricity in our area.

The area urgently needed a doctor because the witch doctors could not solve people's problems. A twelve-year-old boy came to me with his right leg ripped open from knee to hip by a wild boar. I applied pressure to stop bleeding. Since no antibiotics were available, I put sulfa powder into the wound and sealed the wound with tape. The wound needed to be sutured. Being the rainy season road travel was impossible. I told the father to take his son in a boat to Nan.

"I can't pay," the father insisted.

"You have to, to save your son," I responded. Then I said, "I will pay for the trip."

The father accepted the money and took his son to the witch doctor, who cut the wound open and filled it with water buffalo dung. The boy died of septicemia (blood poisoning).

In another crisis case, a local midwife was helping a young girl trying to deliver her baby. The body of the baby was delivered, but the head was still in the womb. I looked in the medical text my father and sister had sent. I learned the situation had two possible explanations. The baby could have hydrocephalus in which the head is too large to come through the birth canal. The second possibility was the mother had twins.

The mother did not have a second baby. The baby's head was a large mass the size of a mid-size watermelon. The baby was dead and to save the mother I had to penetrate the baby's skull through its mouth to reduce the size of the head so the baby could be delivered. Dorothy sterilized an ice pick and warmed cloths in the oven. I put on gloves and inserted the ice pick through the baby's mouth penetrating the skull. Water gushed out, and the bones in the head came together. The baby's head came out. The mother still was in extreme danger with a high fever. I gave her sulfa pills. Gratefully, she recovered.

These cases dramatically illustrated the critical need for a doctor. We prayed for ten years for a doctor, so the missionaries untrained in medicine could pursue the goal of translation and evangelism instead of medical interruptions.

As I continued to pray, a strong impulse and persistent irritating thought came to mind, "You have to be the answer to your own prayers!" How ridiculous if I had only five years to live. Yet, the message that I was to be the answer to my prayers kept being reinforced to me.

Dr. Kraisri was a Thai amateur anthropologist who was also a cabinet minister in the Thai government. He may have been the most politically influential man in Chiang Mai. He visited us seeking our help in contacting the most elusive tribe in Nan Province, the Mrabri. These jungle nomads, known locally as "Spirits of the Yellow Leaves," were an extremely primitive tribe in our province. This tribe had no home or village. They used palm fronds as shelter. As soon as the leaves turned yellow, they believed they could be found by the spirits, so they moved on. I put him in touch with this tribe, and he encouraged them to settle in villages.

When Dr. Kraisri saw the large numbers of patients gathered on our veranda and noted our frustration in trying to deal with their ills. He suggested that I consider attending the new medical college in Chiang Mai. This was to be a cooperative effort between the Thai government and the University of Illinois.

“I personally know the Dean," he said. "Dr. Boonsom Martin is the son of an English father and Thai mother. He is a graduate of an English medical college and specialized in tropical medicine. I will give you a letter of introduction.”

This was soon followed by visits from Dr. Jim Steiner and Dr. McDaniel. Arriving at separate times they helped me go through the card files I kept on patients I had seen. Both doctors said I had a gift for diagnosis and treatment and urged me to apply to the Chiang Mai Medical School. They armed me with letters of recommendation.

Not wishing to face the daunting task of medical education with a limited life expectancy, I went down to our provincial capital of Nan to speak to the Provincial Health Officer. "Is there any possibility of recruiting a Thai doctor to set up a clinic in Pua?" I asked.

He replied, "I cannot think of any doctor who would want to live in Pua. Besides I have heard of the good medical work you are doing in Pua, so why would you need a doctor."

"Because I am a guest in your country and I am technically violating your laws by practicing medicine without a license."

"Nobody is going to arrest you for doing good deeds."

"But I am a Christian, and our Bible tells me I must obey the law of your country."

"Then you must go to the medical college in Chiang Mai!"

Reluctantly, I concluded that the Lord wanted me to make an appointment to see Dr. Martin at Chiang Mai University. I decided to explore my chances of being admitted to medical school. The night before the appointment I stayed with missionary friends at the Overseas Missionary Fellowship (OMF) Guest House.

I wanted them to pray for my interview with Dr. Martin. As we prayed together, I determined that God would have to orchestrate the outcome of the interview, so I did not take the letters of recommendation with me. Still I hoped Dr. Martin would reject me.

Dr. Martin was courteous but somewhat stern in his demeanor. I explained to him the situation in Pua and my reasons for going to medical school. He peppered me with questions.

"How old are you?"

"Thirty-two," I replied.

"We will not admit students over age twenty-five."

"Are you married?"

"Yes, with three children."

"You should know that Thai universities do not admit married students. It is either a degree or a spouse. You can't have both."

"Are you a Thai citizen?"

"No, but I have a permanent visa as long as I don't leave Thailand for more than eleven months."

"Sorry, but we have no provisions for admitting foreign students. What is your educational background, particularly in mathematics and science?"

"Twelve years ago I completed a Bachelor of Arts in Biblical Studies with only a semester of biology."

"That's no help," he said, "You can see why I cannot admit you: 1. Too old, 2. Married, 3. Not a Thai citizen, and 4. Inadequate academic background."

I breathed a silent prayer, "Thank you, Lord. Now I can go back to teaching and evangelism."

As I rose to leave, I thanked him for his time. "Since you cannot admit me as a student when you graduate doctors will you please send a doctor to our area?"

"Wait a minute. Come back here. No Thai doctor would want to live in Pua, 'the Siberia of Thailand.' Government service does not even go there. It is a place for exile or detention."

When I started to leave, Dr. Martin, said, "Come back. I know you want to do this because of your love of the Thai people and no one else will go to Pua. If you can go back to the United States and take all the pre-medical requirements in math and science with no grade below C, I will waive all the rules and admit you as a student in our medical college."

"What do I have to take in eleven months?"

"General chemistry, organic chemistry, physics, comparative anatomy, embryology, advanced algebra and trigonometry."

"You expect me to take all these in eleven months?" I gasped.

"That's the deal," he replied with finality.

The next big hurdle would be to find an accredited college in the United States that would allow me to take twenty-two hours of math and science in an eleven-month period.

I wrote letters to several colleges and universities asking to be admitted to complete these required courses within eleven months. Communication was slow. It took weeks to receive the replies. Polite answers came back which could be summarized in three words. "Are you crazy?"

Finally, two letters arrived which offered a glimmer of possibility. Goshen College, Dr. Steiner's alma mater said they would work with me to try to get me through the required courses in the available time. Wheaton College also responded.

The director of admissions at Wheaton College in Illinois wrote to this effect (not an exact quote.)

> *"Normally we would dismiss your request as an academic impossibility. However, being married to the daughter of Thailand missionaries, I know something of the country and its medical needs. My wife is the daughter of Margaret Landon, the author of the book, Anna and the King of Siam [from which the movie The King and I was derived.]*
>
> *We have a four-week concentrated course in General Chemistry at the beginning of the summer that covers a year's credit. Your mornings would be devoted to lectures, and the afternoons to laboratory assignments. If you can make a grade of B in this course, we will allow you to enroll for the regular school year."*

When Dr. McDaniel, an alumnus of Wheaton, learned of my tentative acceptance, he said, "If you can get through the tough pre-med courses in Wheaton, nothing in medical school can stop you."

The spring of 1963 was a flurry of activity. In May, I was to go to Jerusalem, Tel Aviv, and London to do further research on the plants and animals of the Bible. As stated in chapter 3, the need for surgery in Bangkok to remove my kidney stone, which would have derailed our schedule, was averted. Immediately before the surgery began, I passed the kidney stone. We proceeded with our planned schedule. In New York, I finished *Plants and Animals in the Bible: A Translator's Workbook* (American Bible Society, 1963). While still in New York, we met with Dr. Greenspan who examined our daughter, Grace.

Study Questions

1. In his book *The Circle Maker*, Mark Batterson wrote, "One dimension of *thinking long* is *thinking different* and prayer is the key to both. Prayer doesn't just change circumstances. Most importantly, it changes us. It doesn't just alter external realities. It alters internal realities so that we see with spiritual eyes.....It enables us to see beyond our circumstances, beyond ourselves, beyond time. Is there something you have prayed for "many years?" What is the current situation?
2. Read Ephesians 1:17. When did Paul stop praying for the church in Ephesus?
3. Read Luke 18:1. What instructions did Jesus give to his disciples about prayer?

4. Have you ever prayed for God to send someone to help your friend or family member, only for Him to reveal that YOU are the one He wants to use? Were you eager or reluctant to be used by God?

5. If you were told you only have five years to live, how would you want to spend the time you have left?

6. Garland could not immediately see how it was possible to get admitted to medical school, then to complete a very strenuous schedule of courses in a very short time period. But God orchestrated putting the right people in the right places at the right times. Do you think this was a miracle?

7. Read Matthew 19:26 and Jeremiah 32:17. Discuss this statement: The more impossible it seems, the more God is glorified by doing it!

Chapter 8

Financing Medical Education

Proceeding from New York City, we stopped at Charleston, West Virginia, where my father was superintendent of a psychiatric hospital. Then we journeyed to Chandlerville, Illinois, where Dorothy and the children would stay with Mom Dyson, Dorothy's mother, during my four-week chemistry course at Wheaton. We were thankful that the children had the opportunity to become acquainted with grandparents and other relatives in West Virginia and Illinois.

I took a bus to Wheaton with one extremely heavy suitcase. From the bus station to the college campus it was quite a struggle. Thankfully, an athletic young Wheaton College student relieved me the last few blocks. I arrived at the registrar's office with less than one hundred dollars.

They offered to reduce my payment if I would operate the switchboard and the front door of the dormitory building. These duties interfered with my studies but led to what I considered to be some divine appointments. The roommate assigned to me was Jim, a medical student who had come to take a summer class at Wheaton. He came from a Christian family but had lost his faith as a student at Yale University. He tried to engage me in mocking arguments about my faith.

Finally, I said, "Jim, if you are correct in your assumption that there is no existence after physical death, I still have lost nothing. My faith has given me purpose, direction, and joy throughout this life, plus the hope of a joyful eternity. On the other hand, Jim, if you are wrong, you have not only forfeited the joy brought by faith in God but sentenced yourself to eternal torment." We had no further arguments.

By the time I had paid my registration fees, I had only $35 left. My first evening on desk duty several students stopped by with questions or just to chat. Among them was a young student from Australia named Graham Roberts. He had come to Wheaton hoping to prepare himself for missionary service in the Far East. He was quite troubled at being unable to meet the financial requirements to continue at Wheaton College.

That evening at my bedtime prayers I was startled by the strong impulse, "Give $10 to Graham Roberts!" What a ridiculous thought! But, as the impulse persisted, I quietly went to Graham's room and slipped the $10 under the door. That left me with one $10 bill and three $5 bills to survive the next three weeks.

The next afternoon in class our instructor announced that a certain amount of money had been found under a lab stool. If the owner would report the amount recovered and the location of the lab stool correctly, the money would be restored. I was not aware of having opened my billfold, so I felt it could not have been mine. During the noon hour, I checked my campus mailbox and found a check from a totally unexpected source for $20 -- double the amount I had given Graham Roberts.

As I opened the billfold to put in the check, I was aghast to discover two $5 bills were missing. When I reported this to the instructor, he stated that the money had been found under my lab stool and restored it to me. I suddenly felt wealthy with my $45, the amount I had after finishing my registration.

In the following mail was a check from the American Bible Society for $50. This would be enough to pay a required advance for fall tuition if I passed the requirements in my chemistry class. Again, during my evening devotions the unwanted message came, "Give the $50 to Graham Roberts."

In reluctant obedience with the $50 in hand, I knocked on Graham's door. After I had knocked repeatedly, a red-eyed Graham appeared at the door. He embarrassedly stated that he had been on his knees praying that God would provide the required funds to remain at Wheaton. Graham Roberts and his lovely wife Frieda graduated from Wheaton and went as missionaries to the Indonesian island of Sulawesi (Celebes).

The next mail contained a check for $150.00 from a fellow missionary in Thailand--three times the amount I had given to Graham Roberts. These incidents confirmed two of our convictions:

1. You cannot outgive the Lord.
2. God will provide the needs of those who faithfully look to Him.

Eighteen students enrolled for the intensive General Chemistry/Quantitative Analysis class. At age thirty-three, I was by far the oldest member of the class. My first week in the class I felt lost in a clueless jungle of scientific jargon. My previous exposure to chemistry was in a 1947 high school course before the dawn of the atomic age. The week concluded with a written examination that I flunked miserably, breaking the grading curve.

A brash nineteen-year-old pre-medical student, Phil Olsen, accosted me after the exam. "What's an old Geezer like you doing in this class? How did you do on the test?"

Through gritted teeth, I explained my purpose in studying chemistry and admitted my failure on the test. "Why don't you let me come to your room and tutor you?" he exclaimed. "It could help both of us."

I found living quarters for the entire family just one block west of the campus. An older two-story house had been converted into two apartments usually occupied by missionaries. The owner required no down payment.

The Mortensons occupied the upstairs apartment. Carl Mortenson, a missionary pilot, was in the process of inventing and building an airplane that could safely land on a small jungle or mountainside airstrip. I sent for my family, and we moved into the downstairs apartment. The Mortenson family matched ours with three children. Eddie and Banjel (Evangeline) were younger than Geoffrey and Corinne, but the children enjoyed playing together.

Phil Olson came over nearly every day to tutor me in chemistry. He was especially fond of Grace Eileen, and they would slap hands while Phil would exclaim, "All right!" At nine months, Eileen (the little girl who would never talk) spoke her first words, "All right!"

With Phil's tutelage, chemistry began to make sense. On the second weekly exam, I made a grade of C. At the beginning of the week I had gone to the instructor telling him that I was considering dropping the class since I was totally baffled by the class material. He urged me to stick with the class. "You are working hard and it takes time to readjust to academic life. I am sure you will be able to work up to a passing grade."

My instructor did not know, and I was not about to tell him that a passing grade was not enough. It would require a grade of B to continue my pre-medical studies. To shorten the story, I aced the next two exams and garnered an A in my lab experiments, giving me a B- for the course.

With some apprehension, I went to see Charles Schoenherr, the Director of Admissions. "You told me if I made a grade of B, I could enroll for the fall semester. Will you accept a B-?"

The director smiled, "Can you pay the advance fee for the fall semester?"

"I have exactly the right amount," I replied.

Mr. Schoenherr then told me that in looking at the fall semester schedule, there was no way I could fit in Advanced Algebra and Trigonometry classes. "If you can find someone to tutor you, we will give you credit for the courses, if you can pass the exams."

A new challenge loomed, finding someone to tutor me in the math courses. Mathematics had always been a weakness. Algebra and geometry had significantly lowered my grade averages in high school.

We attended the Christian Church of Glen Ellyn and I mentioned my dilemma to some of our friends at the church. "Why don't you let Chuck tutor you?

This surprised me. Chuck (not his real name), a learning-challenged young man had been unable to attend a regular school. He was a savant, a genius in mathematics, even though unable to learn other subjects. Chuck was brought over to my house by his parents. Amazingly he communicated the math concepts in a way I could understand.

Churches and individuals who had supported our mission work gave generously and we were able to pay our monthly rent and buy groceries. However, one congregation cut off their support, stating that they wanted us to continue tribal evangelism, not to get involved in social work like medical missions. The Christian Church in Naperville picked up the slack and supported us through the remainder of our years in Thailand.

During the summer, I visited churches that had supported us. I bought used textbooks and studied ahead on my fall subjects. The Glen Ellyn Church was constructing a new building, and I was able to go out summer evenings and lay bricks.

Because of the extra care required for Grace Eileen, Dorothy was unable to work outside the home. A gentleman from the Glen Ellyn Church took her and Grace to doctor appointments. The generosity of Christian friends allowed me to pay my tuition in full. Dorothy enrolled Geoffrey and Corinne in the Holmes Elementary School.

The tremor in my hands continued to be a challenge in my lab work, but I cannot remember spilling any reagents (chemicals) or breaking any test tubes. One afternoon in Comparative Anatomy, the news of President Kennedy's assassination stunned our class. The next day in chapel we had a truly memorable memorial service presided over by Dr. V. Raymond Edman, president of Wheaton College, and Dr. Hudson Taylor Armerding, college provost.

We were overcome by the kindness and friendship of the staff and students at Wheaton. At 6:00 a.m. every weekday, several of us met for prayer with Dr. Edman on the top floor of the old administration building. These sessions provided a precious time of sharing and intercession and set a God-centered tone for the day. Dr. Edman's many years as a missionary in South America gave him a wonderful perspective for global evangelism as he led Wheaton College.

A group of students surrounded us with their encouragement and support. Many of them were pre-medical students. These included Phil Olson, Dale Nelson, Carol Wagner, Roland Kawano, Mike Noyes and others, whose names I cannot recall.

January 1964 brought some memorable events. The Glen Ellyn church building had been completed except for a few odds and ends, including the baptistery heater. Eight-year-old Geoffrey decided he wanted to be baptized and did not want to wait for warm water. So on a January day his cold baptism became part of an unplanned family tradition. In March 1915, my father was baptized in Nebraska's Elkhorn River with ice chunks floating down the stream. My father baptized me in April 1937 in a lake at 14,000 feet elevation in the eastern Himalayas. Snow covered the surrounding peaks. Corinne continued the tradition in a cold mountain stream on Doi Suthep near Chiang Mai in 1965.

At the end of the fall semester, I mailed my grade report to Dr. Boonsom Martin in Chiang Mai Medical School. He wrote a warm reply anticipating my summer enrollment in medical school.

Before the beginning of the second semester, Dean of Students, Richard Gross sent me a letter stating that a friend of Wheaton College had endowed a special scholarship for someone preparing for medical missions and that my grades made me eligible. The letter included an application form.

I started to fill out the application form, but these words stopped me, "I hereby request . . . ." Would this be a violation of our promise never to ask people for funds to do the Lord's work?

I decided not to send in the application. A few days later I received a phone call from Dr. Gross, "We have not received your application yet." I made an appointment to talk with the Dean. I explained that through the experiences of Hudson Taylor and George Mueller, as well as my parents' experiences as independent missionaries in Tibet, Dorothy and I had resolved not to appeal to human sources for financial support.

Dr. Gross responded, "I respect your decision, and I note that your tuition has already been paid." The next day after I had made my decision not to apply for the scholarship, we had received enough money in the mail to pay for the tuition.

February 1964 presented a new challenge. An alarming letter from Dr. Martin came stating that the Committee of Medical Education had overruled him. Chiang Mai Medical School could not admit me after all. "We hope you can be admitted to an American medical college and come out and help us after you graduate," he concluded his letter.

Shock! Dismay! Disappointment! This could mean that I would spend at least five years away from the people, languages, and diseases in the area where I had planned to work. Although tempted to give up, I remembered the stone walls God had already led us through.

I barely had time to register for the MCAT (Medical College Aptitude Test) which all United States medical colleges required for entrance, but I made the deadline. After taking the

MCAT, I sent applications to six medical colleges. Rejection letters tend to come back faster than acceptances. The first four responses to my applications were rejections.

Some of the responses: "Anyone who by the age of thirty-four has not decided what to do with their lives lacks the requisite stability to be a medical doctor." And "We have had sad results from admitting candidates over age thirty. The few who succeeded finished in the lower one-third of the class, often by the grace and mercy of their instructors."

Following the rejection letters I received acceptances from the University of Nebraska Medical Center and Hahnemann Medical College in Philadelphia. With heavy hearts, we began plans to move to Nebraska in the summer.

In March came another bombshell from Thailand. Dr. Martin wrote that the Committee on Medical Education had reversed itself. If I could be in Chiang Mai by May 24, I would be allowed to enroll in their medical college the following week.

What followed was a mad scramble to meet with each of my instructors and ask for permission to finish the course work and take my final examinations three weeks early. The Wheaton semester ended mid-June.

Most of my instructors willingly accommodated me. Dr. Spradley, my Physics instructor, went through the remaining assignment and excused me from those he felt were not relevant to medical school. He allowed me to write the examination in his office.

At the other extreme, my Organic Chemistry instructor was very stringent in his requirements. Affectionately, students referred to him as "The Bear." He was so exacting in his assignments that we approached the examinations with fear and trembling. He was reputed to have said, "I have diverted more premedical students into the Baptist ministry than to medical school."

He gave me a key to the chemistry laboratory and insisted that every chemistry experiment be completed before I would be given credit for the course. After the day's class work, I went home for supper and a brief family time. Then it was off to an all-night stint in the laboratory. In April, I learned to live basically without sleep--important training for future years.

In early May, President Edman invited our family to his lovely home. Having lived in a primitive mission field, the Edmans understood the difficulty in getting good quality clothing for growing children. The Edmans had collected a five-year supply of clothes for our three children.

On our final Friday in Wheaton, I collected my grades for the semester to carry to the medical college in Chiang Mai. That evening the pre-med students and other friends staged a carry-in food party in our apartment. The next morning we boarded a Japanese Airlines plane at O'Hare Field for out flight to Bangkok via Tokyo.

As we descended to the stifling heat and humidity of Don Muang airport in Bangkok, the pilot gave us his final greeting with his Japanese accent on the intercom,
"Ladies and gentleman. This is your captain speaking. On behalf of Japan Air Rines, we thank you for *frying* with us. We hope you have had a good *fright*."

The flight to Bangkok had nearly depleted our funds. We had a warm welcome to the Christian Missionary Alliance Guest House, where they charged us the minimum. I flew up to Chiang Mai to take my grades to the medical school and find out if they would admit me without advance payment. Going to the registrar's office, I inquired how much I would need to pay.

She glanced at a list of names and said my name was not on it. Pulling my file she informed me that a college in Illinois had paid half my tuition through medical school. The Thai government had matched it because I would help the Thai people.

I believe the college in Illinois was Wheaton College although the Chiang Mai registrar was not free to give me that information. This fact makes me conclude why I have never received a financial appeal from Wheaton.

The registrar stated, "You will need to pay $100 each year for cafeteria fees." By the grace of God would it mean that I could enroll and graduate from medical college debt free?

Study Questions

1. Garland's friend, Jim, did not believe in life after death, so in just three sentences, Garland laid out his answer. Read aloud the response to this argument. How would you put this in your own words for an unbelieving friend of your own?
2. Imagine having very little money and yet being nudged by the Holy Spirit to give it to someone else who was in need. Would your first response be "Really, God? Are You sure?" or would you put your trust in God's provision without hesitation?

3. Read Ecclesiastes 11:1. The 21st Century King James Version reads like this: "Cast thy bread upon the waters, for thou shalt find it after many days." How does this verse (in any translation) fit Garland's story about giving money to Graham Roberts?

4. A second surprise check arrived which Garland said confirmed two of their convictions. What were the two he listed?

5. A friend suggested Chuck might be able to tutor Garland in his particularly challenging math subjects. He was a savant – someone with extraordinary mental abilities in a particular area yet having developmental issues like "Rain Man." Garland said, "Amazingly, he communicated the math concepts in a way I could understand." Do you think it was *more* than amazing – perhaps even a miracle provided by God?

6. Read Matthew 6:31-32. Share how these verses might encourage someone facing financial difficulties.

Chapter 9

Surviving Medical School

I hastily rented a house in Chiang Mai which proved to be unsuitable for our family's needs. The stairwell opening on the second floor did not have a protective railing around it. Grace Eileen never crawled, but moved about the house by rolling. Dorothy had vivid memories of a younger sister, who was permanently brain damaged by falling down the stairwell at age two.

Several irrigation ditches ran through our property. Also, a badly diseased old dog, suffering with arthritis, partly blinded by cataracts and covered with itchy mange came with the property. The constant groaning and scratching touched our hearts. We went to the property owner and requested permission to put the dog to sleep. She readily granted our request.

We checked with an internal medicine professor at the medical center asking how we could put the animal to sleep with minimal pain. He instructed, "Fill a syringe with adrenalin and inject into the fifth intercostal space with a long needle. The adrenalin will stop the heart almost instantly."

He gave me a filled syringe and I proceeded with my mission of mercy. The feeble animal did not resist my ministrations. The adrenalin missed his heart and entered a network of small blood vessels.

The dose of adrenalin suddenly energized the dog. His eyes brightened; the hair on his back bristled. He was excited but did not know why. With a deep roar, he rushed out the front gate and headed for Red China as fast as his legs could carry him. We found his body about two miles away. "At least he died happy," a neighbor commented. I learned that dog anatomy is not like human anatomy.

We relocated to a safer house in a better location. Our back gate opened into the yard of Chiang Mai Children's Center where our older children would go to school. Dorothy taught there which covered the children's tuition.

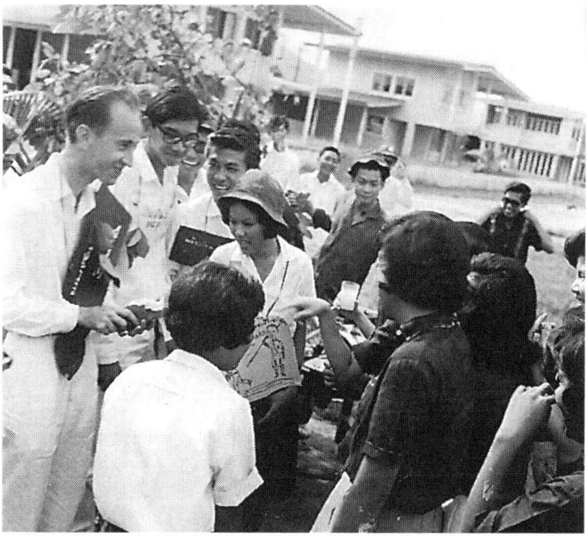

Students curious of the only white student in a university of 6,000

Geoffrey and Corinne attended class with the children of fellow missionaries, diplomats, and Illinois professors of the medical center. Long-term friendships developed from these classroom contacts.

Another bombshell! Dr. Yongyut, Dean of Students, called me to his office and told me I would be required to stay on campus at the men's dormitory during the week with only weekend visits to home and family. I found it difficult to accept this news gracefully.

Not having been through a cultural orientation, I committed a terrible *faux pas* my first day in the cafeteria. I took my tray and sat down at a table with four other students. Frosty silence met my attempt to be friendly. Presently, three of them got up and left. The remaining student spoke sternly, "Freshmen

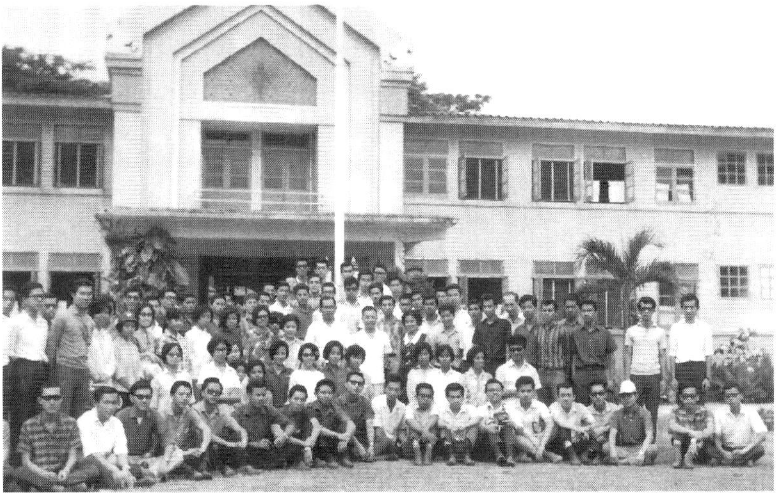

Student Body in front of Chiang Mai Medical Center

students are not allowed to sit at a table with seniors. I am the senior RA at the dorm. Your penalty will be to clean all of the latrines on all three floors for a week."

How should I respond to this embarrassing discipline--*humiliation* or *humbling? Humiliation* could lead to resentment, grudge-holding, and future reprisals. *Humbling* meant a graceful acceptance of the penalty and provided diligent effort for the assigned task. I chose to be humble and put in my best effort.

Students using the facilities could not hide their amusement at seeing the American newcomer on hands and knees scrubbing the plumbing and floors. On the other hand, I sensed growing respect as I performed my duties cheerfully and with no resentment.

The formal initiation of the freshman class included a Buddhist religious ceremony where all were supposed to worship a Buddha image. Of the sixty-four students in the class, four of us were not Buddhists--one an avowed atheist, a Hindu man, a Catholic woman, and myself. Thankfully they did not pressure us to participate in the Buddhist ceremony.

An early encourager of mine, Dr. Arun, Professor of Anatomy, began her life in a household in the canals outside Bangkok. This remarkable woman's brilliant mind led her through a series of scholarships to a Ph.D. in anatomy at Duke University.

She assigned a cadaver to each group of three or four students. I was assigned three of the sixteen female students as lab partners. Dr. Arun solemnly counseled us on our responsibility to the cadavers,

> *These people who donated their bodies to medical science may be the most important teachers in your medical*

> *education. From them, you will learn the name and location of every organ, every blood vessel, every muscle, every bone, and every surface area on the human body. At the end of the class we will have a memorial service to honor these donors.*

The students took these words to heart with no joking or horseplay involving the cadavers. Although Dr. Arun liked to argue creation versus evolution with me, I will forever be indebted to her for the many ways she encouraged and helped me through my freshman year.

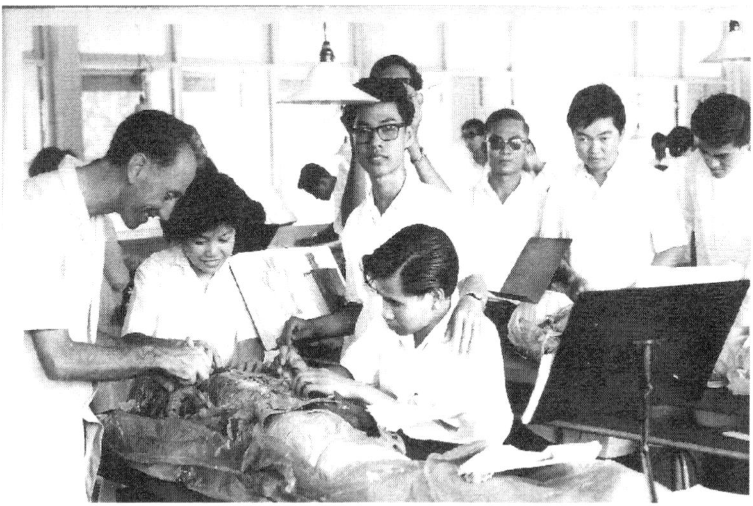

"The people who donated their bodies to medical science may be the best teachers in your medical education"

Living in the dormitory proved to be a blessing in many ways. Being totally immersed in the Thai language from dawn to late night helped me in my future communication. My roommate

Sonpong also encouraged me. Near mid-semester Grace Eileen came down with a severe case of encephalitis and Sonpong requested to be assigned to her case under the supervision of her physician. He spent much time talking and singing to her. Late one night I tiptoed into her room to find Sonpong curled up beside her.

I found it frustrating that the school did not give out grades. They warned me that medical students past age thirty would face challenges to their physical stamina and mental acuity that could well lead to failure.

I prayed that God would keep me out of the lower third of the class for His glory, not for my ego. I experienced an additional challenge in the fact that most lecturers spoke in the Thai language. I wrote very slowly in Thai. We worked out an exchange that I would share my notes on the English language lectures with Thai students, and they would share their notes with me.

Instead of grades, the year-end evaluations listed students in these categories: Pass, Repeat, or Fail. Two students flunked out and three were forced to repeat. Thankfully, my name did not appear under Repeat or Fail.

At the beginning of my second year, Dr. Yongyut told me I could live at home as long as my grades were in the upper third of the class. If my grade point average fell below that, I would need to move back to the dorm. I should also stay in the dormitory on the eve of examinations or when on hospital duty.

The Thai people love squid (calamari) in all its forms. Late on dorm nights when I finished my studies, I would open my door, put some dried squid on my electric hot plate and roast it. The aroma of roasting squid brought numbers of students to my room. While we feasted on squid, I had the opportunity of informally sharing the gospel. Squid evangelism paid off as Bible studies began and have continued through the years.

When we returned to visit the university thirty years later, the Bible studies were continuing. Medical, nursing, and other students have been won to the Lord and continue serving Him in ministering to their countrymen.

In the incident described earlier in the book, my tremor stopped and my hand-eye coordination became normal my first day of assisting a surgical procedure on a living patient. With my newly gifted abilities, I relished the opportunity of working in the emergency room and the surgery theater.

Hospital workers dubbed one of the most frequent injuries seen in the ER as the "Honda Syndrome." Motorcycle riders, most without helmets, clogged the streets of Chiang Mai.

A young man dressed in the homespun blue of a rice farmer was brought in with head trauma incurred in a collision with a telephone pole. I was a proctor for some underclassmen observers. They all understood English when spoken slowly and enunciated clearly. X-rays of the accident victim showed a linear skull fracture of the parietal bone. I explained this to the students when the patient piped up in cockney English, "So, I got a crack in me head, eh, doc?"

I will never forget my first solo delivery. For the patient in her late thirties, it would be her eleventh child, but her first hospital delivery. She didn't want a twelfth child, therefore she needed a tubal ligation. Examination showed her to be dilated about seven centimeters. Immediately following this examination she started pushing.

"Don't push yet," I counseled. "It's not time." The patient answered sarcastically, "How many babies have you pushed out, doctor?" On the next contraction, I caught a healthy baby boy with a powerful set of lungs.

Memorable incidents and dramatic learning experiences filled each semester of medical school. Recounting these would sidetrack from the purpose of the book. I formed strong friendships with my Thai classmates that continue to this day.

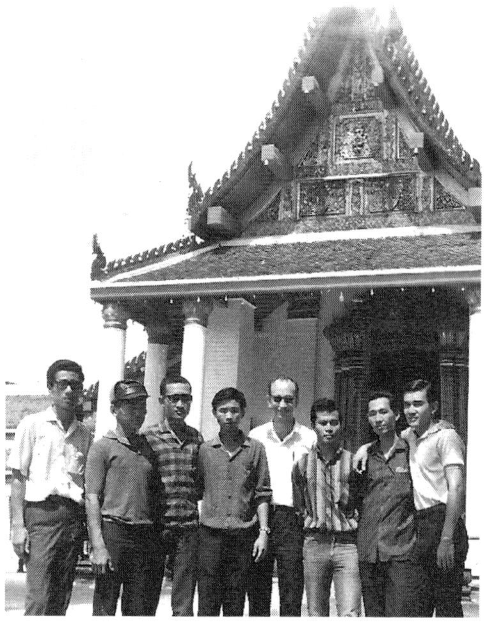

Garland with medical college classmates before Buddhist temple

My fluency in the Thai language progressed to the point that I thought in Thai. Dorothy told me that I would talk Thai in my sleep. I was pressed into service to be a United Nations type interpreter for a large international medical conference in 1968. I gave simultaneous translations of all the lectures. All the participants wore earphones. The Thai participants heard the English lectures in the Thai language. English users heard the

Thai lectures instantly in English. I also translated questions and answers for the audience.

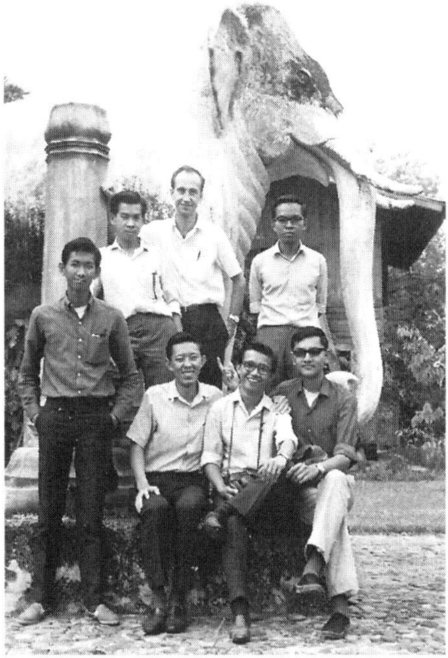

Garland with medical college classmates at 13th century capital of Thailand, Sukhotai

Finally, graduation time came. On a hot day in March 1968, His Majesty King Phumiphon Adunyadet flew up from Bangkok to confer our diplomas to us. His Majesty had a keen interest in medical education. His late father, a royal prince, had a medical degree from Harvard. His mother, the Princess Mother, also had a nursing degree from Harvard.

While we sweltered in our graduation gowns, His Majesty and other dignitaries sat under an awning. Parents of the graduating class sat in a special shaded area. Since my parents were unable to fly to Thailand for the ceremony, C. W. and Lois Callaway served in *loco parentis.* Since I was the only married student, Dorothy and our children got to sit with the class parents.

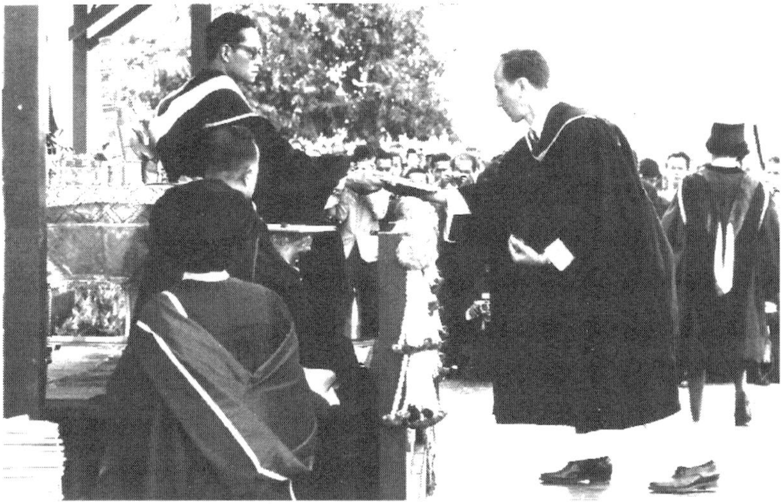

Garland receiving his diploma from His Majesty King Phumiphon Adunyadet

My classmates carefully instructed me in how to receive the diploma and coached me in royal terminology. One was not to use common terminology in addressing royalty. Princess Sunanta, one of my classmates, and others carefully drilled me on the posture and words to use should His Majesty choose to speak to me. Thankfully he did not. I experienced a dreamlike quality in realizing that four and one-half years after starting pre-med, I was a doctor!

Thailand had five medical colleges. All the graduating seniors had to take the same standardized examination. A few days after graduation, I received a letter from the Ministry of Health. The letter read:

> *Congratulations in being among the top ten medical graduates in Thailand. It is a pleasure of the Royal Government to award you a full scholarship for a Ph.D. in any of the medical sciences in Europe or America, provided you sign a contract to return and teach in a Thai Medical College.*

The generous offer overwhelmed me, but I declined because my mission was to serve the spiritual and medical needs of the tribes in Nan Province. I feel a hesitancy in relating the academic honors, but all glory goes to the One who enabled me. As a chorus from my youth goes:

> *He's done so much for me*
> *He's done so much for me*
> *How can I do less*
> *Than give Him my best*
> *And live for Him completely*
> *For He's done so much for me!*

Following graduation, I entered a rotating internship at Suan Dok Hospital affiliated with the medical college. I started the mornings as a phlebotomist drawing blood on all my patients, thankful for the healing of the tremor in my hands. Doing blood smears and cultures provided excellent training for a future of starting a hospital in a primitive area. I learned to distinguish between different types of malaria.

Intestinal parasites were very prevalent in the rural areas of North Thailand. Each species had a different treatment, so it was crucial to make accurate diagnoses of the stool specimens.

The patient's private zoo might contain tapeworms, pinworms, hookworms, flukes, amoeba, or roundworms.

I found laboratory work fascinating, but it did not compare to the joy of being an instrument of Christ's compassion to the multiethnic patients at the hospital. In the course of the year, I used five different languages in hospital rounds.

One exciting day a planeload of wealthy Danish tourists crashed a few miles from the hospital. One crew member died in the crash, but all the passengers survived with various degrees of trauma. Overjoyed to be treated by an American doctor, the Danes loaded us with gifts, including exotic and expensive foods. It seemed bizarre to be feasting on caviar, kippered herring, rare cheeses and pastries in our humble missionary home. "You prepare a table before me in the presence of my enemies" (Psalm 23:5).

During the internship, I had numerous experiences that would not have been likely in an American hospital. Traffic accidents, blood feuds, animal attacks, and injuries from construction gave opportunities for trauma surgery. During the internship, I performed brain surgery and vascular surgery.

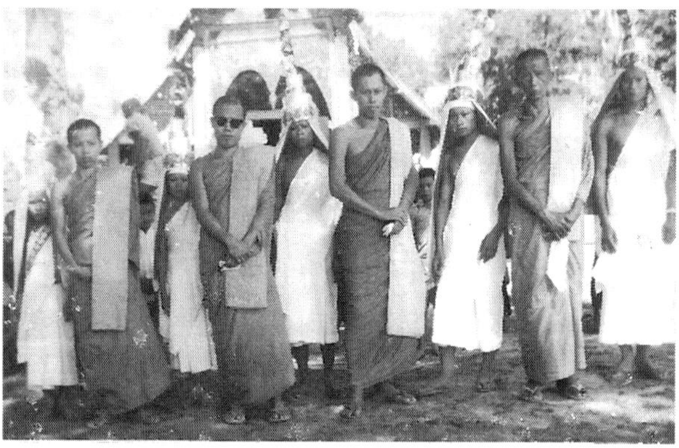

Monks visited and received health checkups

Dealing with epidemics of rare infectious diseases, unknown in the Western world, provided valuable preparation for practicing in the hinterlands. Anthrax is a disease of many faces. *Cutaneous anthrax* comes from skin contact with a diseased animal. The resulting skin ulcers readily respond to antibiotics. *Pulmonary anthrax* rapidly destroys lung tissue. A bloody, frothy cough precedes death in most cases.

We saw two epidemics of *intestinal anthrax.* Dozens of victims came to our hospital. Despite vigorous antibiotic treatment, no patients survived. This disease is caused by eating the raw meat from an animal that died of anthrax.

In spite of the benign sub-tropical climate and abundance of fruits and vegetables in northern Thailand, the people experienced a great deal of malnutrition at that time. Starving and malnourished children filled an entire ward in Suan Dauk Hospital. Some of them had been abandoned by their parents. Nurse Dorothy Sterling adopted a starving three year old who had never been loved and was still not speaking. Little Sharon thrived in an atmosphere of love and good nutrition. Sharon Sterling went on to graduate from a prestigious university and is now a psychologist living in New York.

Study Questions

1. When told he could not live with his family, Garland "found it difficult to accept this news gracefully." Families are a great source of encouragement especially during challenging times, and leaving Dorothy to tend to three young children on her own must have been heart-wrenching. On a scale of 1 to 10 (1 being "no problem"

and 10 being "ready to throw in the towel") how would you have accepted this news ..... gracefully?

2. Look for at least four ways living in the dormitory proved to be a blessing for Garland and his family. Do you see any miracles on your list?

3. Being penalized after an embarrassing freshman mistake, Garland had a choice to make: should he respond with humiliation or humbling? What would be most peoples' human instinct? Which did Garland choose?

4. While his situation was short-lived – only one week – many problems cut much deeper and last much longer. Betrayal by somcone you trust. Abandonment by family. Victimized by false accusations. Have you been punished for something that was not your fault or that you did not deserve?

5. Read 2 Corinthians 12:9-10. How can someone be weak and strong at the same time?

6. C. S. Lewis said, "Humility is not thinking less of yourself, but thinking of yourself less." After overcoming all the odds and proving wrong all those who said Garland would never become a doctor, he was still hesitant to accept the academic honors. Why?

7. Read Jeremiah 9:23-24. Of what should we boast?

Chapter 10

Medical Service in the Green Bug

During our first twelve years in Thailand, the only vehicles we owned were bicycles. Arriving in the rapidly growing city of Chiang Mai for medical school, it became necessary to have a car. The purchase of a new vehicle was out of the question financially, partly due to import duties. I learned that a professor of dentistry at the university wanted to sell her Volkswagen Beetle in order to purchase a larger car for her family. Since I was a poor medical student, she lowered her asking price. The car was an ugly bilious green color, but the finish and interior were in excellent condition. The doctor had neglected to tell me that the brakes were gone.

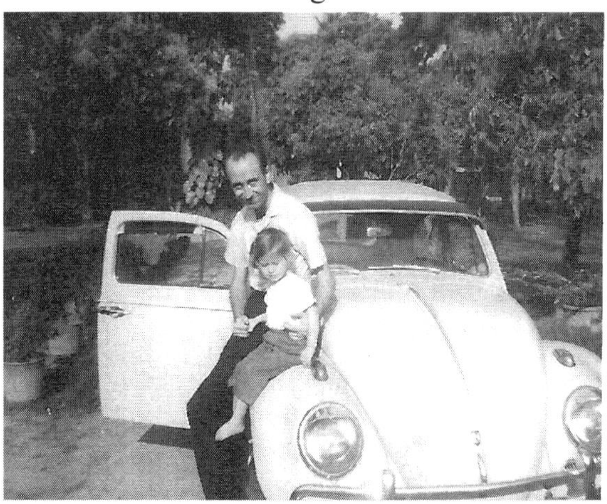

Garland and Grace with the Green Bug (1964)

The drive from her home to the hospital was uneventful until I turned into the circular drive in front of the main hospital building. I saw a bevy of happy laughing nursing students waiting along the drive. I tried to slow down and to my horror discovered there were no brakes. To avoid plowing into the students, I headed for the curb with noisy grinding of gears.

The students turned to stare at the noisy stop. I heard one of them remark, "The American student drives just like American drivers in the movies."

I was the second student to own a car. One of my classmates was the son of a wealthy Chinese merchant. He had taken his pre-medical studies in England and spoke fluent English with a British accent. His father had given him a car to use in medical school.

Our two cars were pressed into unexpected service our second year. One of the gynecology professors was a former ballet dancer and conceived the astonishing idea of having the medical students stage a ballet. My duties were two-fold:

1) I was to be assistant choreographer by adapting a tribal legend to modern dance. (What would the supporting churches think if they found out their missionary was choreographing a ballet??)

2) The other student and I were to use our vehicles to transport a visiting Bangkok ballet troupe to and from their hotel.

I chose a Lisu tale I had heard in childhood as the plot of the musical. With the help of photographs and actual observation of Lisu festivals, we set local tailors and seamstresses busy producing Lisu costumes for the entire cast.

The medical students and professional ballerinas danced well together and the ballet was an immense success. After each performance we transported the professional dancers to their hotel.

One evening my fellow driver failed to show up, and I needed to transport the entire troupe. I told them to wait inside the theater and I could transport them in multiple trips.

"No, no!" they insisted, "We will all get in your car now." I stood aghast as thirteen giggling ballerinas piled in one-on-top-of the other into the Green Bug (I did not contact the Guinness Book of Records to see if I had set a world record for transporting dancers in a VW Beatle).

After repairing the brakes initially, I cannot recall any further trouble the Green Bug gave us. Often I left for the hospital at 6:00 a.m. before the kids were up and arrived home after 10:00 p.m. when they were in bed. It grieved me that Dorothy had to function much of the time as a single parent.

On the weekend I was not on call, we would load into the Green Bug and take an excursion into the countryside. March and April are the hottest months in Thailand. On the upper slopes of Doi Suthep overlooking Chiang Mai, the air was refreshingly cool. Some of the mission groups had vacation cabins.

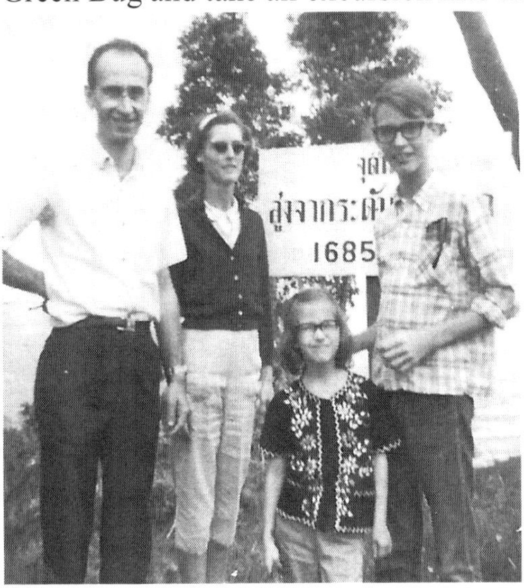

Upper slopes of Doi Suthep overlooking Chiang Mai

Sometimes we would rent one of these cabins for a weekend. If possible, I would leave my medical textbooks behind but take our Bibles, board games, and Agatha Christie mysteries. Trail hikes and playing in mountain streams gave added fun. No slope seemed too steep for the Green Bug.

Some Sundays I preached in area villages. Driving to villages that had no all-weather roads the Green Bug had to bounce along oxcart ruts avoiding buffalo wallows and stumps. Once we ascended steep slopes to a tribal village. The trail had been widened for elephants to pull logs.

As I pulled into the village, some of the tribesmen shielded their eyes staring into the sky. When they realized that the motor noise was not a plane, but the first automobile to enter their village, there was a lot of astonished laughter.

After a busy morning at the hospital, I was entering our driveway one day when the rearview mirror showed an American neighbor running behind the car yelling and waving his arms. "Hurry, hurry!" shouted Mr. G., "My car won't start and my wife is about to deliver our baby!"

The shouting brought Dorothy outside, and she climbed into the Green Bug along with Mr. G. Being definitely in advanced labor, we assisted Mrs. G. into the car and ignored all speed limits in our dash to McCormick Hospital.

"Pant! Pant! Don't push! Don't push!" I shouted as we careened toward the hospital. I dreaded the thought of a delivery in the back seat of a Volkswagen. We pulled up into the ER ramp at McCormick Hospital. ER personnel rushed a cart out, and we were able to load Mrs. G. on the cart before she delivered.

As the internship drew toward a close, I fell into a period of deep depression, probably as a result of unrelenting fatigue and stress. It was then the Lord sent a ministering angel in the person of Mr. Chuck Weeks.

Chuck Weeks, a Missouri farm boy, came to Thailand as a missionary with New Tribes Mission. Not only did he minister to the tribespeople in the remote village to which he had been assigned, but he also had a ministry of encouraging discouraged missionaries.

Chuck spent several days with us sharing Scriptures and patiently listening. By the time he left, the depression had lifted, and I was ready to return to battle.

As the internship came to a close, I wrote to the Department of Surgery at the University of Nebraska Medical Center applying for a straight surgery internship. At the time my father, Dr. Norton Bare, was teaching on campus at the Nebraska Psychiatric Institute and my younger sister, Maribel, had recently completed her residency in internal medicine and cardiology. Dr. Joel Johnson wrote an encouraging letter and said he would arrange a program focusing on trauma surgery.

During the early days of the Vietnam War, a young U. S. Navy doctor observed the chaos that the war was bringing upon the hill tribes. Dr. Thomas Dooley wrote some best-selling books including, *Deliver Us from Evil* and *The Night they Burned the Mountain*, describing the horrors of the situation. His dream was to return after the war and build a hospital. Sadly the young doctor died of malignant melanoma before the dream could be realized.

His friends formed a foundation in his honor to build a hospital bearing his name. The site chosen for the Thomas A. Dooley Memorial Hospital was the old French Fort Carnot on a hilltop overlooking the Laotian town of Ban Houe Sai. The location was across the Mekong River from Thailand.

The structure of the old fort was not conducive to an efficient hospital. The location was precarious, less than one hundred miles from Red China and surrounded by bands of Pathet Lao terrorists. The flood of casualties overwhelmed the volunteer staff. One of the first doctors disabled himself with alcohol consumption. Another put a bullet through his head. The current medical director was a woman physician.

I wrote her that I was finishing an internship and would like to work under her in an externship in trauma surgery before returning to the United States. She wrote a congenial letter welcoming me.

We loaded our family of five and a month's supply of clothes and bedding, plus my medical equipment into the Green Bug. Overloading was simpler in the days before seatbelts and child restraints.

We traveled to Chiang Khong where a ferry would take us across the Mekong to Laos. Dorothy and the children got out of the car. I drove the Green Bug up two planks onto the ferry. Going uphill I could see the planks so I was not particularly nervous about driving onto the boat.

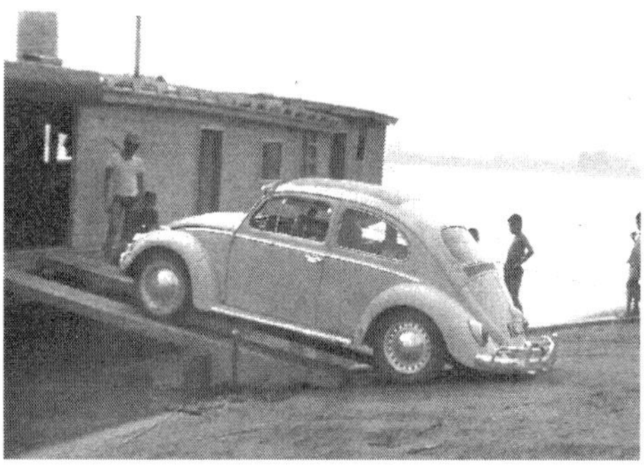

Driving the green bug onto the ferry across the Mekong

On the far side, however, it was a different story. I broke into a nervous sweat as I realized I could not see the down sloping planks. I asked one of the boatmen how deep the river was in case I missed the planks. "More than five meters," he replied. With intense prayer, I crept down the planks with a boatman on the shore guiding the wheels.

...an off of the ferry

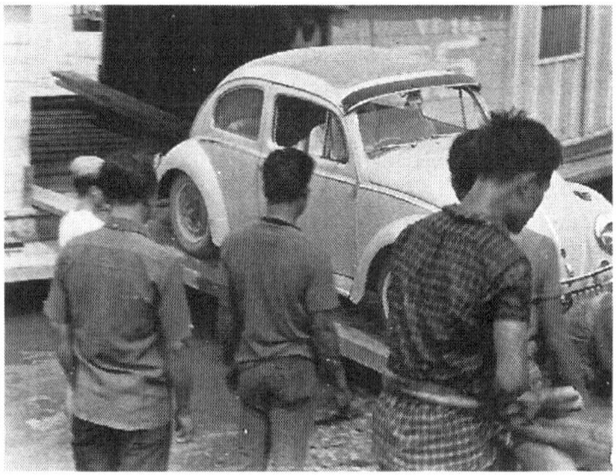

We got through immigration and customs quite easily and proceeded up the dusty street to the hospital. Accustomed to jeeps and military vehicles, residents turned their heads when the little Volkswagen passed by.

Arriving at the hospital, we were greeted by Midge, one of the American volunteers on vacation from her job as a stewardess for Pan American Airways. She was volunteering as a nursing aide. Her cheerful personality brightened many tense days.

Midge delivered the bombshell. "You are now the doctor in charge of the Tom Dooley Hospital!" The doctor who invited me had panicked and absconded. Instead of doing an externship under an experienced doctor, I was suddenly the "boss guy" sadly inexperienced in hospital administration and many of the medical challenges.

Shock number two--we could not drive the disabled hospital jeep until we replaced a broken part. The Green Bug would have to serve as hospital ambulance until we could replace the defective part.

I met the rest of the very interesting staff, nearly all women. Sister Carlotta and Nancy were the nurses. Sister Carlotta was on leave from her convent in Georgia. Nancy Lynch was a nurse from Boston and a lapsed Catholic. Jill was an X-ray tech from Ireland.

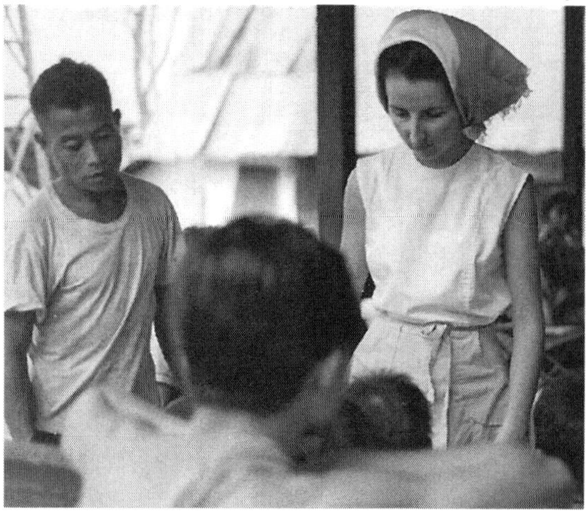

Nancy with patients at Dooley hospital

The rest of the staff were Laotian aides. Midge was a Jill-of-all-trades helping out where needed and spreading cheer when things became gloomy.

We unloaded the Green Bug and spread plastic sheeting in the back to receive injured patients. Workers leveled the hilltop above the hospital to serve as a helipad. When the helicopter clattered overhead, I drove the Bug up under the rotors and loaded the patient with difficulty into the cramped "ambulance."

The first surgical challenge was three small girls, ages four and five, who had picked up an "iron pineapple." When the grenade exploded, the little girls ended up with mangled hands and shredded faces. Fortunately, the hospital had a plentiful supply of tiny sutures with attached needles.

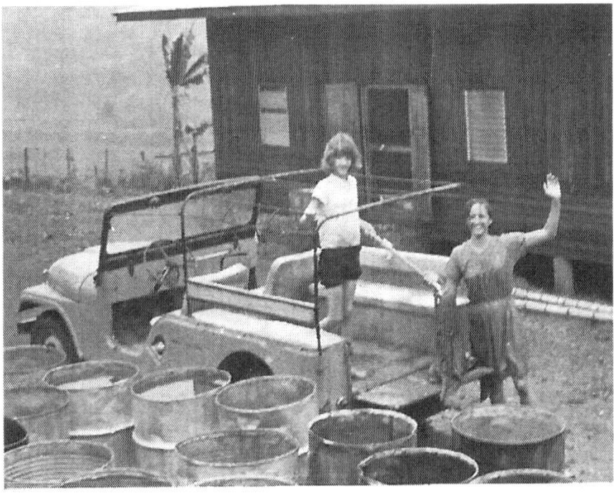

Corinne and Midge with Dooley Hospital water supply

Far into the night we labored under the hot lights. Sister Carlotta administered the anesthetic. Nancy Lynch assisted. At dawn the surgical team retired briefly while Midge monitored the little patients. We kept the little girls for four days, the minimum time required for suture removal.

I had prayed that there would be no significant scarring. A little girl's face is particularly important to her future. Nancy showed me how to remove sutures with a scalpel rather than scissors. The little girls bravely endured the long process of removing dozens of stitches. There were pink lines where the wound edges had been approximated, but NO SCARS! Was this a miracle?

Next, we faced two difficult surgical challenges. A mother and two teenage children were shattered by a land mine. By tribal custom, they were walking single file through the jungle, the boy leading the way, followed by the mother and older sister. Apparently the mother had stepped on the mine and died instantly. The blast shredded the boy's backside. Thankfully, a Filipino army surgeon stopped by and I assisted him in repairing the lower bowel. The girl had shrapnel wounds of the face, breast, and thighs and was permanently blinded. It took hours to repair the wounds.

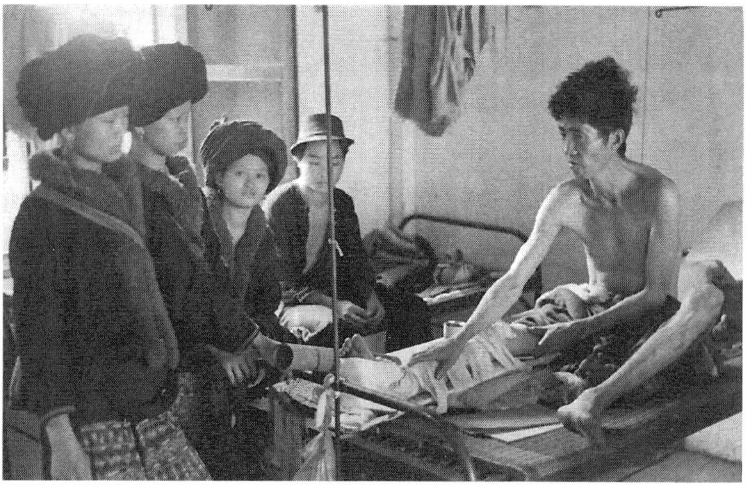

Dooley hospital patient from Mien tribe

A man came in with a distended abdomen. A stone blocked his bladder. We drained about two liters of fluid from his bladder before going in and removing the stone. I was deeply grateful for the Filipino surgeon who "just stopped by."

Patients came to the hospital requiring surgical procedures I had never seen. Dorothy was pressed into service. We brought a music stand into the operating room to hold the surgery manual. While Dorothy turned the pages, I "cook-booked" the operation. During a difficult hernia repair, Dorothy nearly passed out. So Jill took over the page-turning.

Missing equipment complicated our problems. They brought in a nine-year-old boy who was dying of diphtheria. A thick white membrane in the back of his throat blocked the airway and the boy was turning blue. I needed to do an emergency tracheostomy to bypass the blocking membrane, but the hospital lacked the correct size tracheostomy tube. With a pair of forceps I was able to remove part of the membrane. We hastily constructed a steam tent with some plastic sheeting, a hot plate and a kettle of water. While the water boiled, Dorothy, fourteen-year-old Geoffrey and twelve-year-old Corinne fanned the steam toward the boy's nose and mouth. I gave him an antibiotic injection.

My services were needed elsewhere, so the other family members took turns managing the steam tent. By morning the boy was breathing normally, and my family could go to bed. The diphtheria patient went on to a full recovery.

An oxcart brought a fourteen-year-old boy with rabies to the foot of the hospital steps. He was starving and dehydrated. The other name for rabies is hydrophobia meaning "fear of water." At the sight or sound of water, the throat muscles lock in a painful spasm. Along with this goes a strong urge to bite.

I picked up the emaciated boy and started up the hospital steps. Part-way up he pleaded, "Put me down, doctor, or I will have to bite you." I proceeded up the steps and he bit me on the shoulder hard enough to leave blood stains on my shirt. He started sobbing, "I did not want to bite you, doctor, but when the 'Biting Spirit' seizes me I have to bite."

Light bothered him, so we placed him in a dark corner away from other patients. IV fluids and Valium helped ease his discomfort and I tried to share Christ with him. He lived two more days.

Some young boys were brought in, smoldering from a phosphorus bomb. Water will not quench burning phosphorus, so we prepared a potassium permanganate solution. Geoffrey spent most of the night swabbing the wounds to stop the spreading burning.

Government forces captured a Chinese Communist soldier and brought him into the hospital. With badly infected wounds, antibiotics would not stop his slide toward death. As I tried to share the message of Jesus with this intelligent youth, he countered with arguments for communism. "I know we will win," he said, "but I am sad about one thing. When I die my family will not know, and no one will weep for me."

"I will weep for you," I said softly. That seemed to comfort him. He relaxed, sighed, and was gone. And I wept.

Frantic days were occasionally followed by periods of calm. On evenings when Sister Carlotta was not in the operating room, Geoff would go to her room in the barracks, and they would have long conversations about common interests.

While we were there, townsfolk celebrated the Lao New Year or Songkran Festival. This involved dousing each other with water and making charcoal markings on each other. Some of the volunteer girls wanted to go to a local restaurant. Some other Americans in government service joined them. Corinne

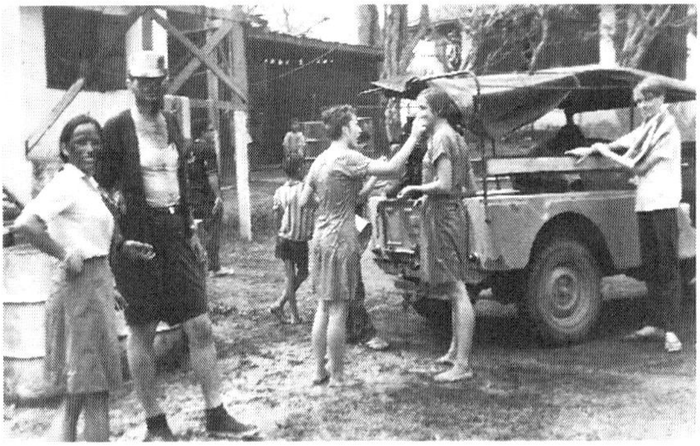

asked to go along and with some misgivings we allowed her to go.

Water and charcoal-decked Songkran revelers

Soon Corinne returned to us in tears. Some of the Americans had become intoxicated. "I can't stand to see my friends get drunk," was her explanation for her early return.

Larry and Verda Peet, OMF missionaries living in Baun Houei Sai, put us in contact with some Lahu Freedom Fighters. They invited me to come up to the Freedom Fighter's Encampment to preach at Resurrection Sunday services. At dawn on Easter Sunday, the Green Bug carried us down to the dock. We engaged a boat to take us several miles upriver to the camp. On the way, a woman on the Thailand side of the Mekong gestured frantically for a ride. Since I had engaged the boat with the provision that they would not pick up additional passengers, the pilot would not pick her up unless I ordered it.

Compassion won out and we pulled over to the Thailand shore and picked up the woman who was on her way to an upriver Lao village.

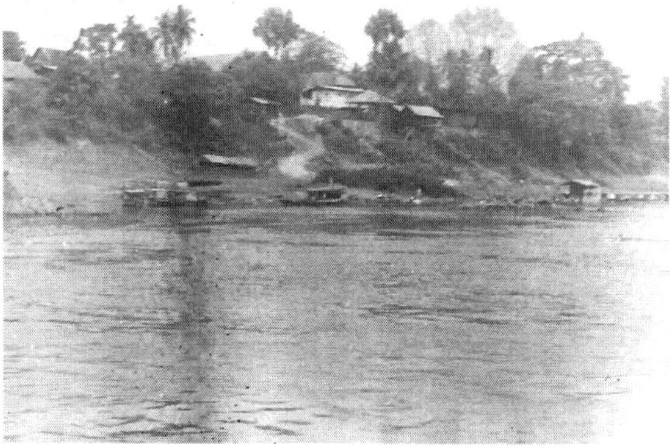

Across the Mekong to Ban Houei Sai, Laos

The government of the country then known as Burma was Marxist and intolerant of Christians. Persecution of tribal minorities, particularly Christians, led to the formation of the Freedom Fighters. We had contact with two of their camps populated by the Lahu tribe. Both camps were inaccessible by road in order to deter the Burmese forces. One camp was on the Lao shore, the other in Burma.

We pulled into the Burma camp about 9:00 a.m. Not having visas for Burma we joined the other illegals for a stirring celebration of our Resurrected Savior. Not speaking Lahu, I preached in the Lao language with a Lahu interpreter.

The singing was uplifting in four-part harmony. A quartet of young warriors sang a stirring rendition of the Jessie Brown Pounds hymn, "I Know That My Redeemer Liveth." We were deeply moved.

Returning to Ban Houe Sai, we discovered that a border incident between Thailand and Laos had closed the border. As soon as we docked, border guards arrested and handcuffed the pilot of our boat for violating the closed border by picking up the woman on the Thai side. They were going to imprison him when I intervened.

"If you are going to imprison him, you will have to imprison me also," I told the Lao border guards. "I ordered him to pick up the lady on the Thailand shore. Neither of us knew that the border was closed." They released the boat captain and fined him a small amount. The Lao guards muttered among themselves. They did not like the idea of imprisoning their only doctor. The Green Bug carried us back up to the hospital.

Later in the week, it was with immense relief that we welcomed Dr. Jim Fleming to the Dooley Hospital. His arrival cut my workload in half. He came from a family practice on the island of Maui and had previous medical mission experience in northern India. He had a congenial personality; the only drawback being the necessity of working through an interpreter.

A few days later I came down with a severe case of dengue fever. I went to work with a fever of 104 degrees Fahrenheit and severe bone pain. The other name for dengue is "breakbone fever." I felt resentful toward my patients because I was sicker than most of them.

Dengue is spread through the bite of the tiger mosquito and is not spread directly from person to person. When Dr. Fleming saw how sick I was, he ordered me to bed with painkillers. Antibiotics do not work for dengue.

A few days later, Dr. Fleming came down with dengue and we reversed roles. When we could both return to work, things ran quite smoothly. One evening when things had calmed down, the doctors and nurses met informally on a screened veranda.

Dr. Fleming jokingly rebuked Sister Carlotta for proselyting. "Sister," he said, "You are trying to make a Catholic out of Geoffrey."

Her reply, "Geoffrey and I both love the Lord and we share that love in our conversations. We also love history and other topics. Neither of us is trying to convert the other."

While Dr. Fleming was ill, they brought in a woman with polyhydramnios--a condition where amniotic fluid may double or triple in volume. This usually occurs when there are abnormalities with the unborn child.

Jill tried to take X-rays, but our small unit was unable to take readable pictures. We decided to do a Caesarean section. The parents calculated that there had been more than eight months of pregnancy. We could not hear fetal heart sounds. Would our suction unit be able to handle the large amount of fluid?

The woman's husband said, "We are very poor. We already have five children. It is hard for us to travel from our village. Can you do something to make sure we do not have more children?" He readily signed a permit for a sterilization procedure.

I knew that another pregnancy with an overstretched womb would endanger the mother's life.

As we set up the procedure, Midge waited with warm blankets in case there was a living child. We said a prayer. As we opened the uterus, there was a gush of fluid that overwhelmed the suction pump and fluid gushed all over the table and sloshed around our ankles.

I lifted out two tiny boys with hydrocephalus, showing no signs of life. Sister Carlotta was administering the anesthetic. As we prepared to close the operating wound, knowing the Catholic views of sterilization, I said, "Sister Carlotta, will you please close your eyes." Hastily, I performed a tubal ligation. The patient recovered well.

One month was coming to an end. Under the capable hands of Jim Fleming and with another doctor coming soon, we felt optimistic about the future of the Dooley Hospital. We had bonded deeply with the staff, and there was sorrow at parting. Midge would be leaving soon to marry her fiancé, an orthopedist in San Francisco.

Sister Carlotta patiently awaiting a tire change

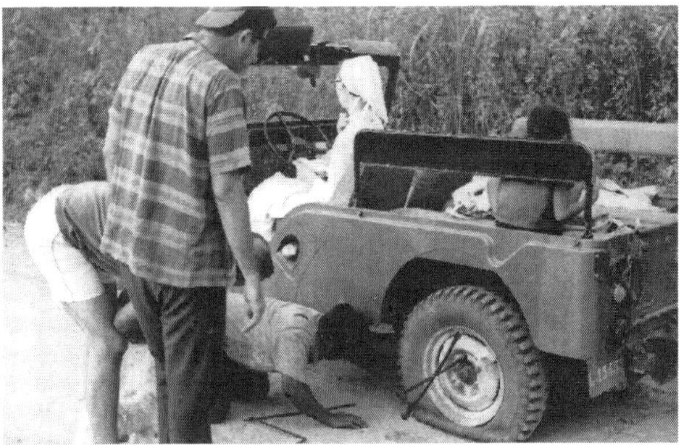

Sister Carlotta planned a ten-day vacation in Chiang Mai the following month. When we asked her if she would like us to arrange a place for her to stay at the convent in Chiang Mai, she replied, "No. I want to stay with you." And we did indeed have a pleasant visit when she came--with no medical stresses.

The Green Bug had no difficulty crossing the Mekong. We began preparations for our summer return for my surgery training in Omaha. What would we do with the Green Bug?

On Sunday mornings in Chiang Mai we would often worship in the independent Thai church led by Pastor Boon Me. One Sunday, Chuck Weeks showed up at church. Chuck traveled by bicycle and bus in his ministry throughout North Thailand. We felt led to give Chuck the Green Bug to speed up his ministry and the little "gospel chariot" carried the Good News for many, many more miles.

Study Questions

1. During a period of deep depression, Garland said, "It was then the Lord sent a ministering angel in the person of Mr. Chuck Weeks. What did Chuck do that made him seem to Garland as an angel?

2. Read Hebrews 11:1. Do you think all angels have white wings and sit around on puffy clouds? Describe the kinds of things that you think angels do, either from Scripture or from popular culture. Which do you think we should believe?

3. Read 1 Kings 19:3-7. Elijah was in the depths of depression after Jezebel plotted to have him killed. He wanted to die. What happened? Have you ever experienced God sending someone to minister to you in a time of dire need?

4. This chapter recalls story after story of people who were saved from certain death due to the efforts of the humble, dedicated medical staff serving the hill tribes. Do any of these stories appear to have miraculous conclusions?

5. It seems difficult to imagine the old Green Bug making the life-saving and spirit-refreshing trips on up and down mountain trails. Why do you think Garland referred to the car as their little "gospel chariot?"

Chapter 11

Provision in Omaha

After returning to Chiang Mai from Laos, we started bustling preparations to move to Omaha, Nebraska for intensive training in surgical skills. After learning about my medical needs in Thailand, Dr. Joel Johnson of the University of Nebraska Medical Center tailored a program for me focused on trauma surgery. This extremely unusual opportunity I attribute to God's undertaking on my behalf. Dr. Johnson later had a distinguished surgical practice in Kearney, Nebraska and became a senator from his district to the Nebraska Unicameral.

Before we left Chiang Mai, we received reports of stepped-up terrorist activity in Nan Province making our return to Pua questionable. Dorothy Sterling, who spent many years as a nurse working with the Lisu tribe in China, hoped to start a work with the Lisu north of Chiang Mai. She suggested I could help her set up a clinic there.

Dr. Richard Buker, a renowned leprosy specialist, had helped the Christian Missionary Alliance (CMA) open a leprosy clinic called the Maranatha Clinic near Khon Kaen on the Northeast Plateau. I met Dr. John Payton, their first full-time physician, at the CMA Guest House in Bangkok. Dr. Payton stated that he would be going to the States for furlough the following year. Would I consider filling in for him at Maranatha for a year?

We had cordial relationships with many of the CMA missionaries and had worked with them in Bible revision and other projects. However, on certain doctrinal issues I felt it would be difficult to work with them. The CMA observed a six month probationary period before baptizing converts who had expressed their faith. We tried to follow the biblical pattern of baptism at the time of conversion.

Soon after we left Thailand, CMA headquarters in Nyack, New York contacted me with an invitation to fill in for Dr. Payton at Maranatha for a year. I declined politely for doctrinal reasons, telling them that our goal was to meet the medical needs of the northern tribes.

As we packed to leave Thailand we received a message from Dr. Fleming informing us that he would like to meet us at the Honolulu Airport. When we arrived there, we found that the good doctor was too busy to come but had sent his pilot in a private plane to pick us up. We flew low giving us a close-up view of the beautiful Hawaiian Islands.

When we arrived in Maui, Dr. Fleming showed us his clinic and then took us on a tour through the spectacular scenery of the island. We enjoyed spending time with him in more pleasant surroundings than Ban Houei Sai. We flew back to the Honolulu Airport in time to continue our trip to the mainland.

Omaha provided a great family reunion. My parents were living there while Dad concluded his teaching responsibilities at Nebraska Psychiatric Institute. My older brother Edgar and his wife Jewel were living in Omaha. Ed was a teacher and counselor in the Omaha public schools and participated in a new church plant--the Twin Cities Christian Church across the river in Council Bluffs. Jewel served as pianist for the new congregation.

The Twin Cities church became our church home during the year in Omaha. Charles Gash was the minister. We could not have dreamed that forty years later Charles would be our neighbor at the Spring River Christian Village in Joplin. While we were in Omaha, Charlie baptized our daughter, Grace Eileen.

We rented a house on Poppleton Avenue within walking distance of the Medical Center. Christian friends helped us obtain a used car. Ladies of one of the Omaha churches taught Dorothy to drive through the busy downtown.

My surgery training began with a week of orientation at the Medical Center. I was officially a straight surgery intern. To be licensed to practice in the United States, I had to take the ECFMG exam, required for graduates of medical schools outside the country. The exam was weighted heavily in favor of American medicine, especially cardiac. Because I did not experience many cardiac cases in Thailand, I was sure I had failed. To my surprise, I passed easily.

The raw experiences of trauma surgery at Suan Dauk Hospital and the Thomas Dooley Memorial Hospital had given me a jump start in practical skills. At the end of the first week, Dr. Musselman, Chairman of the Surgery Department gave us individual evaluations. Glaring at me he said, "Bare, I am kicking you out of the surgery internship!" Shocked silence on my part. "You know too much. From now on I am promoting you to Resident status. If you are able to come back from Thailand for two more years of residency, you will become eligible for board certification.

I developed a profound respect for Dr. Musselman. He sometimes presented a gruff exterior tempered by flashes of mischievous humor. Above all he was a scholar, a consummate surgeon, and he cared deeply for the success of his house officers. He goaded us into excellence.

As a house officer, I received a monthly stipend (my first pay for medical service). Our supporting churches continued to be faithful. One of the surgery residents gave us a car. God was true to His promise to supply all our needs.

My first trauma rotation was at the Douglas County Hospital Emergency Room, a two-block walk from our home. I worked in twelve-hour shifts supervised by the Chief Resident.

One day we received a radio call. The ambulance brought in a DOA (dead on arrival). The middle-aged patient had suffered a heart attack while watching a ballgame. In those days, CPR was in its infancy and ambulance crews were trained as paramedics. My job would be to confirm the patient's death to the family so they could call the mortician.

That evening I was supervising a senior medical student, Steve, who wanted the experience of inserting an endotracheal tube. We had already hooked up an electrocardiogram. I instructed Steve on carefully inserting the ET tube. "Watch for the glottal reflex," I told him, "a spasm at the back of the throat."

"It moved," Steve exclaimed. By this time the EKG showed faint cardiac activity, so I ordered full resuscitation.

The Chief Resident, hearing about it came storming in, "Bare," he rebuked me, "This man was more than ten minutes without oxygen. His brain will not recover. You have resurrected a vegetable!"

The next morning when I made rounds, the patient was propped up in bed. "I want to meet the doctor who said I would be a vegetable," he stated.

When the policemen who patrolled the south side of Omaha would come in accompanying victims of bar fights and traffic accidents, I would often meet them to get a history of the trauma. We served them coffee and donuts while we elicited patient histories. I got to be on a first-name basis with many of these patrolmen.

On my final week at Douglas County ER, I told them that my next rotation would be at Clarkson Hospital learning to do Caesarean sections and deal with obstetric and gynecologic emergencies.

The Benson Church of Christ was between ministers. They asked me if I would fill the pulpit on some Sundays when I was not on hospital call. On the designated Sunday I expected to finish my call duties by midnight Saturday, but a complicated delivery delayed me until 8:00 a.m. Sunday.

In my bloodstained uniform I drove home, took the world's fastest shower, jumped into my suit and tore off for the Benson church, many miles to the north. Then through the rearview mirror I saw the dreaded flashing lights.

As the officer pulled up beside me, he recognized me. "What's the rush Dr. Bare, delivering a baby?"

"No, delivering a sermon. 58th and Miami. Due to be there in 10 minutes!"

"After me, Dr. Bare," he shouted.

I wonder how many Omahans on that bright Sunday morning were startled to see an old Chevy hotly pursuing a squad car with flashing lights and sirens. As we pulled into the Benson parking lot churchgoers stared in open-mouthed astonishment. In later years Benson members loved to recount the dramatic arrival of their guest speaker.

During my Ob-Gyn rotation, one of my patients found out that I was a missionary doctor. She poured out her story to me. "I grew up in a Christian home. If I had followed the teaching of my parents, I would not be in this situation. Can you arrange for my baby to go directly to a Christian family?'

Nebraska law allowed physicians to arrange direct adoption. To the consternation of the social services office at the Medical Center, I did arrange a direct adoption.

I knew the perfect family for the baby. A strong Christian family had a little boy. For medical reasons, they could have no more children. They yearned for a little girl to complete their family. I called them to come to Omaha to get their baby girl.

It was a blessing to deliver a beautiful baby. When the young mother was discharged, representatives of the adopting family would go to her home, sign the required documents and take the baby to her new home. Dorothy and my brother Ed were the chosen emissaries. They were touched by the tears of sorrow of the birth mother and the tears of joy of the adopting family.

The baby grew to be a beautiful and talented young woman who brought great joy and pride to her parents. She attended a distinguished university on a music scholarship. She now uses her talents as a college music teacher and church musician and plans to attend a seminary to refine her gifts for service.

The Omaha Veterans Administration Hospital occupied an imposing tower on South 42nd Street and served as a major landmark in the city. My VA Hospital rotation involved leading and mentoring four or five medical students. Our morning rounds covered nearly eleven stories from the Radiology Department on the lowest level to the surgery wards and suites near the top levels.

I noticed that some of the medical students were getting pudgy, so I banned the use of the elevators. I developed a motto for the students, "Elevators are for the aged and infirm and those who are passively rushing into these conditions." I overheard some background muttering about having to follow "the old slave driver."

Years later while practicing medicine in Lincoln, one of the hospitals hosted a reception for a new neurologist joining a local practice. He recognized me, "I remember you! You were the old slave driver."

Life in Omaha meant different things to each family member. Grace Eileen attended J. P. Lord School located on the Medical Center Campus. This was a specialized school for children who faced physical challenges. My nephew Steve Bare attended before his death from Muscular Dystrophy. Several of Grace's schoolmates had cerebral palsy. Individualized education combined with access to physical and speech therapy guided the students toward a productive life. Another amazing aspect of all this was that we received all these benefits free of charge.

We enrolled Geoffrey and Corinne in Norris Junior High School which was within walking distance of our home. Corinne found a small circle of close friends leading to long-term friendships. The foul language and inappropriate behaviors shocked both children in their first encounter with public school.

For Geoffrey, the year was devastating. His accent, his behavior, and his values were objects of ridicule by his classmates. Bullying made each day one of dread. It was a common experience for missionary kids (MKs) coming from a distant country and different culture. Having had similar experiences as a child coming from Tibet, my heart ached for my son.

Due to a shortage of house staff, I faced an intense work schedule when I returned to the University of Nebraska Hospital. Forty-eight hours of being on call meant that I could not leave the hospital building. A blur of activity characterized each day--surgical procedures in the OR could take place any hour of the day or night. These alternated with outpatient clinics and rounding the inpatient rooms. X-rays and laboratory tests had to be closely monitored.

A room with a cot furnished a place to catch a few winks between cases. Being so exhausted, I slept through one emergency call, but another resident stepped in and handled the case. We had pagers but not cell phones at that time.

I experienced times of congenial fellowship with Christian residents and students. One of the surgery residents, Dr. Richard Bransford, went on to a tremendous medical ministry in East Africa spanning more than forty years as a physician and surgeon caring for children with physical and mental abnormalities. I had opportunities to encourage the Christian medical students. A freshman medical student, Dale Michels was to play a significant role in my life in later years.

One day I was called out of a case conference by an emergency call from New York. It was from the President of the Christian Missionary Alliance. His message said something like this: "The CMA headquarters staff has been fasting and praying about a doctor for the Maranatha Clinic to replace Dr. Payton while he is on furlough. You have turned us down twice, but we are going to ask you to pray about it again and get back to us."

I admitted that I had not given much prayer to the decision. My reluctance to go to Maranatha was not only due to doctrinal issues. In climate and scenery the Korat Plateau in Northeast Thailand is not an attractive part of the country. I would need to learn the Lao Isarn dialect and maybe a smattering of Cambodian to communicate with patients. Leprosy care was not my preferred field.

I agreed to give the invitation more prayer and confer with elders in our supporting churches before calling them back. The elders at Lake Station Christian Church in Indiana and Camp Point (Illinois) Christian Church proposed these terms:

1. I would be free to exercise my convictions on the plan of salvation and baptize believers as soon as they declared their faith and repentance.
2. We would continue to be supported by independent Christian Churches and Churches of Christ and not receive a salary from the CMA.

When the Holy Spirit leads one expects unanimity and our advisers were unanimous in their recommendations. So I should not have been surprised when the CMA leadership readily accepted the terms.

The largest CMA church in Omaha was the Omaha Gospel Tabernacle, housed in an imposing building in the downtown section of the city. Pastor R. R. Brown led the congregation through many years of solid growth. They contacted us to see if we would consent to a sending service before we left for Maranatha.

We were honored to accept. The night of the sendoff, they seated our family at the front of the auditorium. After the singing of mission-themed songs, the pastor and other leaders laid hands on us and offered moving prayers.

As we prepared to return to Thailand, I was asked to say a few words about our mission plans at our final case conference. Dr. Stevenson, a faculty member who had served as a medical missionary in Africa, offered a prayer. Dr. Musselman stated his appreciation that I had remained upbeat through a grueling year.

A retired surgeon, with a daughter married to a Thai national, invited me to his home to pick up some equipment. He gave me a large pack of surgical instruments that could have cost many hundreds of dollars.

The nurses of the surgery department collected dressings, bandages, tapes and baby blankets. When we left for Maranatha we were well equipped without financial expenditure on our part.

Study Questions

1. Due to his unique circumstances, a special program was tailored for Garland to study trauma surgery in Omaha. He said, "This extremely unusual opportunity I attribute to God's undertaking on my behalf." How would you restate this sentence in your own words? Does your sentence include the word 'miracle?'

2. During his residency, a peer gave the Bares a car. "God was true to His promise to supply all our needs." Read

Philippians 4:19. What is the assurance we get from this verse? Do you think the phrase "all our needs" really means ALL our needs? About which of our needs should we worry?

3. Following a complicated delivery that lasted into the morning hours, Garland was running late to preach at a Sunday service. As he sped toward the church, an Omaha policeman whom Garland had met in the ER stopped him, then escorted him with lights and sirens so he could deliver his sermon on time. Would you call this an amazing coincidence that Garland received this help?

4. We love to hear and read about big, flashy miracles that make headlines. Do you think God provides small miracles in our everyday lives? Think of some examples where you were surprised by "a God thing" just popping up in your life.

5. Throughout medical training in Omaha, Garland said "I had opportunities to encourage the Christian medical students." In what ways do you think he encouraged others?

6. Read Matthew 6:8b. While providing for the Bare family in Omaha, God met all their needs in a variety of ways. If God already knows our needs, why do you think we need to ask Him in a prayer?

Chapter 12

The Maranatha Clinic

As we returned to Thailand in 1970, several questions occupied our thoughts.

- How would we fit in with our new fellow-workers?
- Would my recent training in surgery be wasted in a medical practice focused on leprosy?
- What would we do about high school education for Geoff and Corinne?
- How qualified was I to understand and treat Hansen's Disease (the correct name for leprosy)?
- What would Dorothy's role be besides mothering and teaching Grace Eileen?

⌖ ⌖ ⌖

After the initial few days in Bangkok for customs and immigration, we took the train to the Northeast Plateau on our way to the Maranatha Clinic. We passed through Korat, then the chief city of the Northeast. Irene Brock and Honor Warden met us at a small station near Khon Kaen.

The Christian Missionary Alliance (CMA) built Maranatha Village on a well-laid-out plan. Mission staff homes lined the access road on the north side, and homes of the national staff were on the south side. Students enjoyed playing soccer on a large open field. On the eastern edge was the clinic with an open courtyard. Patients requiring overnight stays occupied a long, low building with several rooms.

We moved into Dr. Payton's house. Like the other missionary homes, it rested on "stilts" embedded in a concrete platform. The stilts, in this case, were solid timber supports. The concrete platform served as a garage, laundry area, and a dry play area for the children during the monsoon rains.

Two cobras were spotted in the area. I dispatched one of them, but the other lurked nearby. Grace Eileen and her playmates, Kevin and Kenny Brock, were supervised when they played downstairs.

Speaking of snakes, one of my patients brought us a fifteen-foot long reticulated python. The Lao girl who assisted Dorothy in the kitchen fixed the snake meat into a sour soup flavored with tamarind leaves. We had enough for us and all our neighbors though some squeamish missionaries refused our generosity. Probably all the snakes of Thailand are edible but not quite as delicious as *ngu singh* or lion snake.

Mali Jun, our plump nursing assistant, had a deathly fear of snakes. One day she went over to tidy up the patients' quarters. Just as she arrived at a door, a lion snake crawled out from under the building. A squealing Mali Jun jumped higher than expected for a woman of her proportions landing astride an equally terrified snake that was moving in confused circles. Up and down went Mali Jun. Round and round went the snake. The clinic staff gathered at the windows laughing themselves to tears over the snake dance. Knowing that lion snakes are harmless, our only concern was that the jumping aide would become an orthopedic casualty.

A building across the soccer field from our home housed the Bible School. The School trained students with leprosy to be pastors and church leaders for the many leprosy villages scattered across the Korat Plateau. Dorothy taught classes there under the supervision of Randy Brock.

The Clinic on the east end of the campus was my sphere of duty. Early in the morning patients would start arriving at the clinic building on foot, by oxcart, bicycle, all manner of motor vehicles and even chartered buses.

Som Jai registered the patients. The first eighty patients to register would be our day's quota. We did manage to work in a few extra patients. Those registered gathered in the courtyard, and a Lao evangelist would then present a gospel message.

The Lao Isarn dialect is close to the Thai language. So my patients and I were usually able to communicate, but when we hit a snag, Mali Jun would step in and interpret. Within two to three weeks I was able to communicate without an interpreter.

The leprosy of modern times is not identical with the leprosy of the Bible. But, socially they are the same. Both biblical leprosy and modern leprosy are contagious diseases requiring isolation of the disease victim. Both inspire fear and revulsion in the general population. Some of the signs of the disease described in the Bible are absent in modern leprosy. Likewise, deformities of the face and extremities common to modern leprosy are not described in the Bible.

Rapid mutations in bacteria present a monumental challenge to modern medicine. Soon after an effective antibiotic is formulated, resistant populations of bacteria develop, rendering the antibiotic ineffective. It is quite possible that biblical leprosy has been extinct for a long time and modern leprosy developed fairly recently. Under the microscope the acid-fast bacilli of leprosy are practically identical to the germs that cause tuberculosis.

Even though we were familiar with leprosy in our years in northern Thailand, being surrounded by people with significant deformities of extremities and distorted facial features was initially a shock for Dorothy and me.

Canadian missionary Irene Hearn had served at Maranatha since the community started. Soon after our arrival at Maranatha, I asked her, "How long did it take you to get past the ugliness of the people?"

"Ugly?!" she exclaimed, "These people are beautiful." By the end of the year we could agree with Irene. The joy of salvation and the beauty of holiness far outshone the physical distortions of these dear people.

As mentioned earlier, the official name of modern leprosy is Hansen's Disease. Carriers of the disease resent being called "lepers." There are three forms of the disease--one affecting mainly the skin, another mainly affecting the sensory nerves, and a third with combined characteristics.

During our time in Maranatha, an explosion of knowledge became available about the causes, treatment, and prevention of leprosy. When my father practiced medicine in Tibet, the preferred treatment was an extract of the chaulmoagra tree. This had little effect in most cases.

Following World War II sulfa drugs were the standard treatment, but act slowly. Some highly effective antibiotics were expensive to produce and could cause serious side effects. The dreaded "lepra reaction" occurs when masses of killed bacteria cause a life-threatening condition by releasing toxins into the system. This could be alleviated by administering Thalidomide. The United States banned Thalidomide because of its deforming effects on the embryo in early pregnancy. We were very cautious about using Thalidomide on a young woman of childbearing age.

Two of the older patients met as students at the Bible School. Because of the deforming effects of the disease in their youth, neither had married. They were both in their forties when they fell in love and got married at Maranatha. Then they went to his new pastorate at a village near Cambodia after they graduated. Within a very short time she became pregnant.

I was fearful for the possible complications of a first-time delivery in an older woman with long-term leprosy. I instructed them to return to Maranatha a month before her due date so we could carefully monitor her condition up to delivery.

Fortunately, I was blessed with three highly capable American nurses. Joy Boese grew up on the mission field in Thailand and was fluent in Thai. Her father Harvey Boese was Field Chairman of the CMA in Thailand. Irene Brock was the wife of the Maranatha Bible School Principal and was a fellow Nebraskan. Janet Greenleaf had lived in a kibbutz in Israel before becoming a missionary.

When our patient went into labor much prayer went up. It turned out to be a perfect delivery. Long years of working in the fields had strengthened the abdominal muscles. Leprosy had killed the sensory pelvic nerves. Delivery was quick and painless. The parents named the son of their old age little Abraham. They chose Abraham instead of Isaac because Isaac in Thai means "makes me vomit."

Because of the long incubation period between exposure and the first manifestations of the disease, congregations practiced strict segregation when we arrived at Maranatha. At the communion service in the Maranatha Chapel, well people sat in a separate area from those infected, and we had separate communion trays.

Residents with leprosy were not allowed into the yards or homes of missionaries. We knew of two missionaries who developed leprosy--one in Hawaii, the other in Africa. The Clinic staff showered and changed in the laundry room under the house before wearing clean clothes up to the living quarters.

Research published in 1970 indicated that leprosy is primarily transmitted in two ways, prolonged skin-to-skin exposure and infrequent hand washing. During the hot season Lao parents carry their naked children against their bare skin. First signs of leprosy often appear in their children by age ten. Leprosy is not transmitted by breathing, sneezing, coughing, or body waste.

Armed with this information, I began to relax the strict isolation rules. Wherever Dorothy and I live, we plant a garden. One day I noticed a group of Maranatha Bible School students standing wistfully outside our garden fence admiring the zinnias and marigolds. I went down and opened the gate. The astonished students came into the garden. "Pick any of the flowers you want. Enjoy yourselves," I said. I noticed that each of the girl students returned to their dorm with a bouquet in hand.

Tong Rin was a zealous young minister in a growing village church. He came down with severe jaundice. He could not afford medical care in Khon Kaen, the nearest city, so he came to us. All we could do was give him symptomatic care as we did not have the sophisticated diagnostic equipment we needed. The young preacher's health continued to decline.

One night I was suddenly awake. "Go to Tong Rin," came the strong impulse. No audible voice, but I knew I must obey. Quietly I dressed and slipped outside. A full moon silvered the palm fronds. No sounds in the night except an owl and distant dogs barking. I walked silently toward Tong Rin's door.

"Doctor?" came the weak voice from inside. "I knew you were coming. I was praying you would. I think I am dying. Do you think the Christian people could help my wife and little boys? There is no one to harvest my rice fields."

Several of us dug into personal emergency funds to get him to Khon Kaen Hospital. The hospital surgeon took one look at him and said, "Liver flukes." I assisted with the surgery. When we opened him up, the liver had the appearance of a termite-infested chunk of wood. Hideous fat flukes crawled in and out of holes. The treatment for flukes is quite hazardous containing arsenic. We tried to kill the flukes without killing our patient.

Geoffrey and Corinne were home on vacation from the Dalat School in Malaysia. Geoff and I, along with students from the Khon Kaen Bible School and men from Tong Rin's congregation took hand sickles and got all his rice harvested in a day. Corinne and the other volunteers skillfully bound the stalks into sheaves. By evening, we had all the sheaves delivered to Tong Rin's grain bin. Women from the village would thresh and husk the rice.

My loosening of the segregation rules caused some consternation among the older missionaries. I allowed Geoffrey to play soccer with the Maranatha students. One day a missionary from another province came to visit along with her teenage son who attended school with Geoff. The boy immediately ran out onto the soccer field.

"Mike!" (not his real name) his mother screamed, "Get away from there!"

Corinne enjoyed attending meetings with the Maranatha youth group and quickly made friends with the girls.

⌖ ⌖ ⌖

Upon our return to Thailand in 1970, we hoped to be able to send Geoffrey and Corinne to a high school where they could interact with Christian kids their age. The International School in Bangkok served children of diplomats, military, business people, and some missionaries. Stories of drug use and other forms of misconduct discouraged us from sending them there.

The Dalat School was started in the cool mountainous area of Viet Nam. The Communist invasion of Viet Nam made it unsafe to remain there, so the CMA moved it to the Cameron Highlands of Malaysia.

When we moved to Maranatha, I discovered that my duties would not be confined to the clinic there. I was also to be the doctor for all the missionaries on the Korat Plateau and do school physicals for students at the Dalat School. Those extra duties gave us discounts that made tuition and transportation affordable for us to enroll Geoff and Corinne in the Dalat School. Was it another miracle of God's provision?

The winding mountain road to the Cameron Highlands made Geoff terribly carsick. Once we reached the plateau, Geoff and Corinne were thrilled with the beautiful cool setting of the school. They made friends readily and many of these friendships have lasted through the decades since.

It surprised them that some of their classmates were lukewarm in their faith and bitter toward their parents. CMA mission policy had been to send the children away to boarding school at age five or six. Seeing their parents only a few weeks during school breaks led to resentment, and in some cases, a feeling of abandonment. Their classmates and teachers became their functional family with no cell phones at that time; letters provided the main means of communication between parents and children.

Geoffrey and his new friend Peter Dutton liked to get up at dawn and run five miles. With growing concern about the spiritual state of some of their peers, they decided to conclude their running time with a period of prayer focused toward a spiritual revival in the student body. Then other students, both boys and girls, joined Geoff and Pete in their time of intercession. Soon a spirit of repentance and renewal swept through campus.

Tranquility on the Dalat Campus was short-lived. Communist terrorists were invading the Cameron Highlands. The school would have to move again. The safest new location appeared to be Penang Island off Malaysia's West Coast. From mountaintop to seacoast, the students and staff moved to a beautiful waterfront campus.

The student revival continued, and soon after relocating, several students were baptized in the Strait of Malacca, an arm of the Indian Ocean. We were privileged to go down for Geoff's graduation and rejoice in the spiritual fervor of the senior class.

On trips to Penang, I was able to do school physicals for the students.

One of our fears in working at Maranatha was that doctrinal difference might lead to conflict. However, we all focused on our love for the Savior recognizing that our true enemy was the Evil One. God blessed us with a spirit of love and unity and the missionaries we worked with became lifelong friends.

One of the leprosy congregations near Maranatha was planning a baptismal service and invited me to speak. Knowing that the CMA espoused the Zwinglian view on baptism, I determined that I would not express any opinions. I merely read all the accounts of baptism and doctrinal statements from the Thai Bible substituting Lao Isarn words where they differed from the Thai.

No commentary was necessary. At the end of the service the pastor exclaimed, "Now I see it! Now I see it! I understand exactly what the Bible teaches about baptism!"

Much more could be written about the Maranatha experiences, but to do so would deviate from the intent of this book. But, one more story needs to be told.

In the city of Khon Kaen was a Bible training school for non-leprous students. Frequent business trips were necessary to the city. We always received a warm welcome from George and Edna Heckendorf, resident missionaries who worked with the school. I had also been invited to preach at the city church.

One of the Bible students shared exciting news with us. "My great-grandmother has just been honored by His Majesty (the king of Thailand) for being the oldest resident in our kingdom. She is more than 110 years old. After the rice harvest, I want to take you to meet her."

After the rice harvest, we had to wait a few weeks for the paddy fields to dry. The oxcarts then broke a trail through the fields and the mud walls that surrounded them.

Our student friend showed up with a borrowed Jeep. The Jeep followed the oxcart trail over what seemed to be hundreds of speed bumps before we entered the village. We found the ancient lady seated and happy to greet us.

I addressed her, "Grandmother, I have never had a patient your age. I would be interested in hearing some of your experiences."

"I do not wish to speak of the first hundred years," she replied. “They were years of darkness and confusion. Then my son brought me the good news of Jesus and I stepped into the light. My only complaint is that my eyes have clouded and I can no longer weave."

She showed Dorothy some of the attractive patterns she had woven. She then brought her gnarled hands together in a prayer of farewell. And we returned on the oxcart trail.

Before we moved away from Maranatha, I made an exploratory trip back to Nan Province. Could we return to Nan Province? Could we return to Pua and open up a medical work? "No," said the United States Embassy. "We cannot guarantee your safety." "Yes," said the Thai government, "but only with strict precautions."

Study Questions

1. Working amidst numbers of severely deformed leprosy patients was initially a shock for the Bares, but before long they agreed with the fellow missionary who said, "These people are beautiful." What did Garland say made them beautiful?

2. Read 1 Samuel 16:7. The modern culture places enormous value on beauty and physical appearance. How does the Lord see us?

3. Read 1 Peter 3:3-4. What is of great worth in God's sight in these verses?

4. When Tong Rin, the young minister is their village became ill, Garland was suddenly awakened in the night with a strong impulse to go to Tong Rin's home. Not knowing why, Garland arrived at his door in time to get him to a hospital. Have you had a time when you felt an unusual or sudden urge to call or visit someone without knowing why? What happened if you did or did not follow that impulse?

5. God can speak to us in a number of ways: through His Word, through other people, through music and worship, through circumstances. How can we be most "tuned-in" to hearing from God?

6. Read Psalm 46:10. Why is this difficult to do in our daily lives? Think about what you can do to find quiet time to listen for God's voice every day?

7. The Bares were privileged to meet a woman who was 110 years old during their time at Maranatha. When asked about her life experiences, what was her reply to Garland?

8. If you have made mistakes in your past, committed sins you think can never be forgiven, carried heavy burdens of your poor choices, how would it feel to come out of that "darkness" and into a fresh, new life with Jesus as the Light of the world … and the Light of YOUR world?

Chapter 13

Back to Khon Kaen

A year after we moved away from Maranatha, the Thai churches of Northeast Thailand invited me to come back to Khon Kaen as speaker for their annual convention. The warmth of their welcome was overwhelming.

Hugging was not an acceptable form of greeting in those days. While chatting with some Thai friends, it startled me that a pair of strong arms locked me in a tight squeeze. It was Tong Rin, healthy and sturdy after his near-death ordeal with liver flukes.

A few months later Pah, a young man of the Hmong tribe in Nan Province, asked me if I could take him to Khon Kaen to enroll in the Bible School there. He had never attended school but could read and write in the Thai language. The Bible School accepted his application.

Due to Communist infiltration of the tribal minorities, all tribesmen carried identification cards. Between Pua and Khon Kaen there were at least three border patrol check points. As we neared the first checkpoint, Pah exclaimed, "I forgot my ID card!"

We faced a dilemma. To return to Pua would mean that Pah would miss new student orientation at Khon Kaen. To try to bypass the checkpoints on country roads would be unthinkable.

"Maybe I should hide under my bedroll," suggested Pah.

"No, if they found you hiding, it would heighten their suspicions and you might do jail time," I replied. "We must be open and aboveboard."

We stopped the pickup by the roadside for a time of prayer. Pah's prayer, "Lord, when we get to the checkpoint, please cover me with Your hand and make me invisible."

My prayer, "Lord, we believe it is your will for Pah to go to Bible school to study Your Word. We ask you to take us through the checkpoint safely."

At that time, Thailand and the United States were partners in the war against the Vietnamese Communists. Americans were held in high regard. When we came to the first checkpoint, I showed the officer my U. S. passport. He took no notice of Pah and wished me a good trip.

The officers at the next two checkpoints waved us through without stopping. Probably the first checkpoint had radioed ahead. "I think God made me invisible," Pah said.

At the Bible School in Khon Kaen, Pah became fluent in Thai and adept at handling God's Word. Nearly twenty-five years later when we returned to Thailand, Dorothy and I found Pah at the Hmong church faithfully serving the Lord.

Like thousands of immigrants from Southeast China, Jiem Meng's parents were very poor when they arrived in Thailand. However, with the work ethic and industriousness typical of the Cantonese, they soon worked up out of poverty to relative prosperity.

I have no idea why they chose to live in Uttaradit Province, one of the least desirable of Thailand's seventy-two provinces. Uttaradit had a bad reputation as an extremely hot area. It was the northernmost province of the vast central plain.

Bounded on the north by low mountains, it formed a natural oven as the heat from the plain was reflected back by the slopes. In March and April daytime temperatures regularly soared to triple digits and the nights offered little respite. Only when the monsoon rains swept in during May was there any relief.

The immigrant couple began by selling trinkets and snacks from a cart. They soon accrued enough income to rent a wooden structure in the market. The downstairs became the shop and the growing family slept under mosquito nets in the hot upstairs.

Jiem Meng was their oldest child. He attended the local Thai government school and received private tutoring in the Chinese language. Chinese parents spurred their children to academic excellence. They usually outperformed the laid-back Thai.

Jiem Meng topped his class academically all the way through high school. In the competitive examination for university scholarships, he came in first in the province, winning a scholarship to a prestigious university in Bangkok.

Between high school and college, the young scholar noted an oval patch on his left arm that was paler than the surrounding skin. The oval area stayed dry unlike the sweaty skin surrounding the oval. Alarmed, he consulted a local doctor. The doctor blindfolded him and did a pinprick test that confirmed the dreaded diagnosis - *Leprosy!*

Jiem Meng's parents saw their pride plummet to dismay and alarm. "You cannot stay here," his mother wept. "You could infect the rest of the family. We will pay your train fare to the Christian leprosy colony in Chiang Mai. Missionaries love lepers."

The bitter young man saw his parents for the last time as he boarded the train for the McKean Leprosy Colony. There he heard the message of God's love from staff and fellow residents.

"How can you talk about God's love when he allows my life and hopes to be completely destroyed?" Jiem Meng railed. "I would shake my fist in his face!"

Enrolled in classes at McKean, he vigorously argued against the Bible's teaching. He had an opportunity to study English and became an apt pupil. Gradually the loving warmth of his teachers and caregivers broke down the wall of hostility. He surrendered to Christ. The power of God's love expressed through His Word transformed his bitter heart into a heart aflame for Christ.

Meanwhile, the devastating disease continued its physical destruction. His facial features became distorted. His fingers locked into tightly flexed claws. He lost all feeling in his feet and had to wear special shoes to protect them from destructive trauma.

Thankfully his vision was not affected and he read the Bible voraciously in Chinese, Thai, and English. He held a pencil between the knuckles of the forefinger and middle finger of this right hand and wrote copious notes from his studies.

He moved to Northeast Thailand and worked with the Christian Missionary Alliance. He became a translator of Christian books including the writings of A.J. Tozer into the Thai language. His eloquence as a preacher and teacher put him in high demand for speaking at conventions and evangelistic meetings. Jiem Meng was the most brilliant and articulate Thai preacher I had heard.

Physically, his leprosy was in remission. When I examined him in KhanKaen, I found no bacteria in his skin biopsies. He was what some leprologists called, "a burned- out case." However, the toxicity of years of medicine resulted in early kidney failure.

In 1974, we prepared to leave Thailand. The Christians in the Pua area wanted to have a farewell preaching-teaching convention. They chose Jiem Meng as one of the convention speakers.

We were happy to see him again. He was amazed that he could sleep in our guest room and share meals at our dining table. He had never been allowed to eat or sleep in missionaries' home. "This is a foretaste of heaven!" he exclaimed. "Where there are no barriers."

As he stood up to speak at the convention, he held up the claws that had once been his hands and he proclaimed, "I thank God for the gift of leprosy, for without it I would never have experienced the love and mercy of our Lord Jesus Christ!"

Study Questions

1. No passport would surely present a problem for Pah and Garland at the checkpoints along the road to Khon Kaen. Once they agreed to be open and honest with the guards, what did they do next? How did their prayers differ?

2. Read 1 John 5:14-15. We are to show our confidence in God when we pray, and He hears us if we ask …… how?
3. Read Matthew 6: 9-10. We as human beings want OUR will to be done. But as we present our requests before God, we need to pray for HIS will to be done. Read

Garland's prayer with Pah again. Did he pray with confidence? Did he pray specifically for their needs? Did he pray for God's will to be done?

4. When young Jiem Meng was achieving academic success and winning competitions, life was good for him and his family. What happened that turned their lives upside down? His bitterness caused him to reject God's love and lash out at the missionaries for their faith. What was his question to them?

5. As Jiem Meng's body was becoming more and more devastated by leprosy, what was happening in his spiritual life? What was it that transformed his bitter heart into a heart aflame for Christ?

6. Read Romans 15:4. Everything written in God's Word is there for a reason. Think of someone you know who is living a life filled with hope. Now compare with someone who does not know or who has rejected God's Word and the promise of hope. How do these lives look different?

7. At the end of the chapter, Jiem Meng made a proclamation that might surprise a lot of people. What did he proclaim? How can Jiem Meng's experience encourage you or someone you love when going through difficult circumstances?

Chapter 14

Provision of a Hospital

Several hard questions faced us as we prepared to return to Pua.

- How can a hospital be built, staffed, and equipped without fundraising? People in the United States and Thailand had told us we could never build, staff, and equip a hospital without fundraising.

- How safe is it to move my wife and three children to a combat zone infiltrated with terrorists against the advice of the United States Embassy? The United States Embassy had told us not to go to Pua because of the danger. If we did go, they would not evacuate us. At the end of our time at Maranatha the Thai government said we could go back to Pua under strict rules--no travel at night.

- Can we continue to house and educate tribal children in the hostel without putting them at risk?

These and other questions confronted us as we prepared to return to our beautiful valley. Yet, a blessed calm filled our hearts as we trusted the One who had never failed us.

Before moving the family, I made a quick trip to Nan, our provincial capital, to consult with the Provincial Health Officer. When sober, he was a delightful conversationalist and he was sober the day I visited him. He had strongly encouraged me to go to medical school.

"I am back to start the medical work in Pua as soon as you guide me through the proper steps I will need to follow to get permission to build a small clinic and hospital."

He said, "No."

I responded, "Why? You wanted me to get my medical training and come back."

His reply stunned me, "You don't need to do that. We knew you were coming back so while you were away, we built the hospital. It will be ready as soon as the electricity and water are installed."

"The Thai Department of Health," he continued, "will provide you with staff and medical equipment. We also hope to recruit a Thai physician to assist you."

As soon as I could recover my breath, I responded, "There is a problem, sir. I am a Christian missionary. How could I practice my faith in a government hospital?"

He replied, "It is true that Buddhism is our official religion. We would ask you not to hold religious services in the hospital building. However, if you feel that there are elements of your faith that would be helpful to the needs of individual patients, feel free to share with them."

I returned to Khon Kaen to bring the family back to Pua. Geoffrey and Corinne had returned to school in Penang. We purchased a Mazda pickup in Bangkok. We placed our possessions in the back. Dorothy and Grace Eileen shared the cab with me. The ruts that formed the road from Nan to Pua were in dry season condition. Imogene Williams and our Thai workers had kept the house in good shape.

The Pua residents eagerly welcomed us back and there was high anticipation for the opening of the hospital. I was excited to inspect the building that was located on the hilltop less than two blocks from our home.

The layout of the hospital was convenient. The reception desk faced the front door. Two examination rooms were just north of the reception desk. These rooms also contained the doctors' desks. North beyond the exam rooms were the equipment rooms and the surgical suite. To the south of the reception desk was the ten-bed hospital ward.

Totally unexpected was our first emergency case. Young children riding the necks of water buffalo were a common sight. The young riders guided the gentle beasts through the fields and along bamboo-shaded village lanes. Biting flies tormented the animals and they often tossed their horns from side to side to shoo the pesky insects away.

A nine-year-old girl astride her buffalo was accidently gored through the abdomen by the animal tossing its horns. Her family brought her to the unfinished hospital in shock with a deep abdominal wound. She was in no condition to be evacuated to another hospital. Only two staff members had arrived, a nurse-midwife and an infectious disease tech. Looking through my meager supplies, I found antiseptic soap, surgical tools, and a powerful flashlight.

We hastily draped the surgical table and the nurse-midwife scrubbed the area surrounding the wound. I washed my hands in a bucket of water and donned the sterile gloves. The midwife monitored the little patient's vital signs. The infectious disease (ID) tech held the flashlight. I injected the anesthetic and without a surgical assistant proceeded as rapidly as possible to repair the perforated bowel. The anesthetic would last only thirty minutes. I then inserted a drain, closing the wound; the patient aroused on the last stitch. We had managed to hydrate her with an IV infusion.

An army jeep was available and we evacuated her to the provincial hospital in Nan with the nurse-midwife accompanying her. Much prayer had been offered during the impromptu surgery. With so much potential for infection, we were glad the little girl made a remarkable recovery and returned to school a few weeks later in good health.

When the medications provided ty the Thai government arrived, I noted an inadequate supply of antibiotics. Those that did come were of doubtful origin and potency manufactured by obscure pharmaceutical companies scattered across southern Asia.

I was surprised to receive an invitation from the United States Air Force Base in Udorn, Thailand to come and conduct Easter sunrise services. There was no direct highway from Pua to Udorn so the trip entailed driving a long distance south, then cutting back northeast through Khon Kaen to Udorn. This involved about 400 miles to cover 120 miles of distance. Some of the officers at the base had become acquainted with our work at Maranatha.

I spent the night with missionary friends at Udorn. At dawn we assembled in the base chapel and I preached on the power and hope of the resurrection of Christ. Some of the airmen were scheduled to fly dangerous missions over Laos and Vietnam that day. I asked if I could write down their names so I could pray for them.

The base physicians told me that they were required to dispose of their antibiotics a month before they expired. Could I use them? The monthly shipments solved our antibiotic problems for awhile. We made certain that we used them before the expiration date.

Years later in Lincoln, Nebraska I went with missionary Al Juve to view a replica of the Vietnam War Memorial. I could not hold back the tears as I saw the names of some who had been at the Easter sunrise service at Udorn Air Force Base.

Soon after the hospital was staffed, Dr. David Filbeck and his family moved back to Pua. David was a linguist who pioneered work in the Lua tribe. His wife Deloris was a registered nurse who had grown up in the Blendville Christian Church in Joplin, Missouri.

A young woman named Surang from a tribal group in Northeast Thailand had been trained as a laboratory technician. She was a radiant Christian and felt called to be a missionary to Pua. Although crippled by polio she was a dedicated worker.

Deloris, Surang, and I formed the Christian minority in a largely Buddhist hospital staff. As I recall, there were three nurses, three nursing assistants, and three midwives. The only other men on the staff were the infectious disease tech and the janitor/orderly.

Soon after the Filbecks arrived, the Thai government built a military camp close to their home, nearly a mile west of us. The Pathet Lao terrorists had set up a base on the mountainside about five miles to the east.

All night there were loud exchanges of heavy artillery and mortar fire between the two camps. These shells passed directly over our home and the hospital. It was as though God had placed a protective canopy over us. During the entire war no shells or shrapnel landed on our property.

I knew that although most of my patients professed loyalty to the Thai government, some of them were sympathetic to the Communist terrorists. Several government soldiers had been wounded in nearby skirmishes and others were ill from malaria or typhoid. One section of the hospital ward had been set apart for military casualties.

One day a patient of mine whispered to me, "The Communists are coming tonight to kill all the soldiers. It will be after midnight." I notified the district militia and they sent one soldier to help patrol the front doors.

After discussing the threat with Dorothy, I decided that I must stay with my patients. Unarmed, but conscious of God's protection, I sat between the waiting room and the hospital ward.

The back entrance to the hospital had been barred. The militiaman paced back and forth in front of the main entrance. After 2:00 a.m. he had disappeared.

Just before 3:00 a.m. I saw a few suspicious movements in the shadows beyond the lighted area. I stood up and walked smiling to the front entrance. The intruders melted into the darkness.

The next day all my military patients were transferred to the safety of the Nan Provincial Hospital. It was an immense relief to the night nurse and the entire hospital staff.

I did not enjoy two areas of patient care. Muey Thai is a form of boxing that involves using the feet. Kickboxing has recently become popular in the United States. Knowing some of the long-term effects of repeated blows to the head and body, I deplored the practice and would not have voluntarily attended. However, the government required me to be the ringside physician available to injured combatants.

The second area was the monthly checkups of the prostitutes for sexually-transmitted diseases. A brothel had been set up near the military camp. One of the commanders explained to me that this was necessary to protect village girls from the soldiers.

As the heavily made-up girls came in for their checkups, their sad faces and empty eyes made my heart ache. Surang tried to witness to them for they would not trust the words of any man.

Study Questions

1. Despite the dangers and questions as the Bare family prepared to return to Pua, they felt "a blessed calm." What was the reason for this peace?

2. Read Lamentations 3:20-23. When we are worried and start to get downcast about a situation, what can we call to mind to have our hope restored? In what circumstances does God's compassion fail?

3. Read Hebrews 10:23 and Deuteronomy 31:6. If you believe God will never fail you or leave you to fend for yourself, and He is faithful to those who trust him, do you believe you can experience that feeling of "blessed calm" in your life?

4. Imagine the scene where emergency surgery was being performed on a nine year old girl with serious wounds. No electricity or running water amidst the flurry of activity with the small staff working feverishly to save this little life. What else was happening during the impromptu surgery?

5. Read Jeremiah 32:17, Psalm 46:1, and Psalm 56:3. When things seem out of hand or even impossible, what should we remember?

6. Garland said "we were glad the little girl made a remarkable recovery and returned to school a few weeks later in good health." Thinking of the theme of the book, is there another word you might use for "remarkable?"

7. Those who are not familiar with what the Bible says might struggle when circumstances seem difficult like this surgery, or even hopeless. We need the assurance of God's promises of faithfulness and provision in all situations, and recalling Scripture is of great comfort and help. Yet it is hard to just open the Bible and start reading by yourself. What benefit would you gain by reading the Bible together with a small group of friends? What other ideas do you have to help learn more about what is in the Bible?

8. As war escalated in the area of the hospital, heavy artillery and mortar fire were exchanged all night. The shells passed right over the hospital and the Bares' home, with nothing landing on the property. To what did Garland credit their safety?

Chapter 15

Hospital Case Histories

Western medicine presented a new challenge to the Pua District. Twentieth-century Western medicine confronted centuries of witch doctor's charms and potions, herbal remedies, and rituals. Soon after the clinic opened, a village woman came in asking to see the room where I concocted my medicine. I explained that we received the medicine from America where specialists prepared it.

"If you don't know the people who concoct the medicine, how do you know whether they have magic powers?" She shook her head in disbelief.

Some of the early patients even saw the stethoscope as an instrument of magic. A patient came in by oxcart with a badly swollen knee--so painful she could not stand. I told her I would need to drain fluid from her knee. This would be slightly painful but then give her relief. I anesthetized her knee with a tiny needle. Then with a large bone needle I drained about 100ccs of cloudy fluid indicating an infection. Before we wrapped the knee she said, "Now will you put the magic ear on my knee?"

Stifling my exasperation, I tried to explain to her that there is nothing magic about a stethoscope. "I put it over the heart to hear if it is working properly. I listen to the lungs for signs of disease. I listen to the working sounds of the belly and sometimes in late pregnancy I can hear the baby's heart beating. The stethoscope has no healing powers."

She stared blankly, "I traveled two days for this. Now will you put the magic ear on my knee?" Completely defeated, I placed the bell of the stethoscope on her knee. "There!" she exclaimed, "It feels much better."

After wrapping the knee. I instructed her to find a place to stay in town. I wanted to examine it again the next day before she went home. We were both gratified by the improvement. She said she could stand up without pain. As I wrapped up her knee again and gave parting antibiotics and instructions, she said, "Thank you, Doctor! I will tell all my friends about the magic ear!"

⌖ ⌖ ⌖

Another elderly woman came in from a distant village. "My vision is so cloudy I cannot see the faces of my grandchildren," she said. "Do you have eye medicine to help me see?"

A quick examination showed advanced cataracts in both eyes. "There are no eye drops that can help you see clearly," I told her, "You will need an operation to remove the cloud objects from your eyes."

She replied, "I am too old to have an operation. You must have some medicine that can help me."

The lady was obviously disappointed at the prospect of leaving empty-handed. "I do have some drops that will soothe your eyes when the dust of the road irritates them," I told her. I gave her a bottle of Visine.

A month later she was back. "I want another bottle of that wonderful medicine."

"You mean it helped you see better?" I inquired.

"Oh no, it did nothing for my eyes. So I put some in my deaf ear. There was a loud pop and suddenly I could hear again." Thus I found out that Visine can dissolve earwax, but I have never recommended it for that purpose.

⌖ ⌖ ⌖

Of the diseases, Anthrax was one of the most dreaded we encountered in Southeast Asia. We dealt with it in three forms. The severity depended upon the part of the body involved.

Cutaneous anthrax came from direct contact with an infected animal. It formed chronic skin lesions that could smolder for months. Thankfully, it usually responded fully to penicillin.

Pulmonary anthrax caused painful and rapid destruction of lung tissue. Patients presented with coughing of bloody frothy sputum. Death came from internal bleeding. Early diagnosis and aggressive treatment have resulted in a few cures.

Earlier in the book, I mentioned that while a medical student at Chiang Mai University, we encountered two epidemics of *intestinal anthrax.* Despite intensive treatment, there were no survivors. This form is contracted by eating the raw flesh of an animal that has died of the disease.

One of the favorite dishes of the rural Thai is *larb* consisting of chopped raw meat mixed with hot peppers, salt, and other spices. A dead water buffalo or ox can feed an entire village.

A young rice farmer came to the hospital one day with all the classic symptoms of acute appendicitis. We prepped him for surgery fully expecting a straight-forward appendectomy. Instead, we found a normal appendix in a sea of bloodstained fluid. There were huge lymph nodes and hemorrhagic areas of the bowel.

I called for a sterile tube and sent for Surang to come to the lab. I instructed her to stain a slide and look for "bamboo-stem bacteria." The bacteria which causes anthrax resembles no other. Large rod-shaped bacteria line up in a formation resembling the segments of a bamboo stalk. A time-consuming culture is not necessary. Immediate diagnosis can be made from a blue-staining bamboo-rod formation on a slide.

"I see many bamboo-rod bacteria on the slide," Surang reported. I instructed the entire O.R. staff and Surang to take the utmost precautions because of the contagious nature of anthrax.

We had a good stock of antibiotics at the time, thanks to the generosity of the Udorn Air Force Base. I irrigated the patient's abdomen continuously with a strong antibiotic solution.

As soon as he recovered consciousness, I asked the patient if he had eaten raw meat recently. He stated that a water buffalo had died recently and they had prepared a large amount of *larb.*

I asked district authorities to round up all the villagers who had already eaten the raw meat to come to the hospital immediately. Nearly forty villagers came and received prophylactic doses of penicillin. A deep pit needed to be dug outside the village. The *larb* was to be cooked with careful precautions and dumped into the pit for burial. Anthrax spores can survive for years and we wanted to take no chance.

Our patient survived and none of those who had eaten the raw meat sickened. If I made any significant contributions to medical science, it was in the first cure of an intestinal anthrax case and prevention of a deadly epidemic. But the credit really belongs to the One who guided me through the ordeal.

⌖ ⌖ ⌖

The spraying of villages with DDT in the Pua District more than doubled the survival rate of infants and children in our malaria-ridden area. The population explosion that ensued put considerable economic pressure on young families.
The midwives in the clinic asked me to accompany them on a clinic trip to teach family planning. Birth control pills were relatively new at the time. We did not fully understand their mechanism of action nor could we foresee their long-term side effects. (In later years I stopped prescribing them.)

One young woman with four children under age six stated that they could not afford another child. I explained the birth control packets instructing her carefully to take one tablet at the same time each day.

A few months later she showed up at our outpatient clinic frustrated and angry. "Your pills are no good! I am pregnant again."

"Did you take one every day as I instructed? I inquired.

"I did until they started making me sick to my stomach," she replied "Then, I turned them over to my husband and he took one every day."

⊕ ⊕ ⊕

Xai Suav was a respected leader among the white Hmong tribesmen of the Luangprabang District of Laos. About 1969 he began to experience excruciating headaches accompanied by severe nasal congestion. The symptoms progressed to difficulty swallowing and loss of balance. For the once vigorous tribesman it meant exposure to multiple potions and charms and frequent visits to the renowned shaman of the Khmu tribe. None of these remedies worked. Through the tribal grapevine he heard of the American doctor across the Thai border who could speak the Hmong language.

Xai Suav and his wife crossed the border into Thailand arriving at dusk at a Blue Hmong village. The warmth of the reception he received surprised him. A long-standing animosity had existed between the White and Blue Hmong sub-tribes.

"Welcome! We no longer see you as enemies, but as brothers," the villagers greeted them. They proceeded to share their new faith with Xai Suav and his wife, telling them how faith in Jesus had overcome their life-long bondage to fear of the demon spirits. "Now we have love and joy!"

"Do you think the American doctor can cure my disease?" asked Xai Suav.

"We do not know whether he can cure your disease," they replied, "but he can help you overcome the fear of death. He is the one who led us to Jesus."

The next day Xai Suav came to the hospital. Examination showed that he had a massive tumor behind his nose--carcinoma of the nasopharynx. It had invaded his brain and neck bones. I told him that nothing short of a miracle from God could cure his cancer. Radiation treatment might prolong his life, but it could not cure him.

They opted for radiation therapy desiring some extra time to move their family from Laos to Thailand. I drove them to Chiang Mai and introduced them to the radiologists.

A Vietnamese refugee had constructed a metal roof with windows for my Mazda pickup. It served as a church bus, school bus, family transport, ambulance, and hearse. The new all-weather roads had transformed Pua into a bustling town with electricity and running water.

When Xai Suav and his wife returned from the radiation treatments, they moved to the refugee camp at Paklang, about five kilometers east of our home in Pua. They had nine children. Soon after their return from Chiang Mai, Xai Suav and his wife confessed their faith along with their youngest son Seri who was about nine years old.

`We received a telegram from Penang that Geoffrey and Corinne would be coming home for school vacation in two days arriving at the Nan Airport. By then a Thai doctor had arrived at the Pua Clinic, so I was free to drive Dorothy and ten-year-old Grace Eileen down to Nan to pick up the older kids. The students at the hostel helped me clean and shine the "Blue Bus" for the happy occasion.

After meeting them at the airport, we expected to drive back to Pua in the mid-afternoon. I cannot recall what delayed our departure from Nan, but it was nearly dark when we left.

The terms for our return to live in Pua prohibited driving after dark because of terrorist activity. Now we had no choice but to drive through darkened hills. Flashlights flagged us down as we passed through a bamboo forest. Suddenly we were surrounded by men in combat gear but with no insignias.

"Aha, *farangs* (foreigners)!" they exclaimed. We were unsure whether our captors were government forces or terrorists. As I rolled down the window, their leader inquired, "Who are you?"

"I am the American doctor from Pua," I replied.

"An American? Good! You can repair our truck," they rejoiced. "It is a Ford, made in America."

They did not point their weapons at me as they escorted me to their concealed truck. As we stumbled through the dark, I frantically prayed for Dorothy and the children surrounded by leering soldiers. I also prayed for a mechanical miracle to get the truck started since I am neither experienced nor adept at auto mechanics.

Under the lifted hood of the truck I noted that two of the spark plug wires appeared crossed in the wrong direction. I unplugged them and re-plugged them in what appeared to be the right sequence. I instructed the driver to start the engine. It ran perfectly.

"Chai Yo! Chai Yo! (Hurrah! Hurrah!)," the men shouted as they patted me on the back. "We knew the American could do it!" "Good luck!" they said as they let us proceed. We knew more than good luck was at work.

Back in Pua, Xai Suav and his wife because enthusiastic members of the intertribal refugee church. However, he steadily weakened to the point he could no longer stand or walk. His pain became excruciating.

After clinic hours, I would jump on my bicycle and visit with Xai Suav and his family. They had not had time to learn to read, so I read Bible passages and explained them. Before I left, I gave Xai Suav an injection of morphine to allow him to sleep.

As time went by I wondered what was keeping Xai Suav alive. All body systems were failing, but his mind remained clear.

The Hmong people have a strongly patriarchal social structure, and leadership of the family passes from father to the oldest son. Xai Suav's oldest son had been mentally disabled by childhood encephalitis. The second son had a terrorist bullet lodged in his brain and was functionally disabled. This would leave the fourteen-year-old Pov Li as head of the family.

Pov Li was a brilliant youth. While still living in Laos he had memorized enough of the tribal sagas and traditions to reach the status of "tribal elder." The baptism of his parents and younger brother offended him deeply. Pov Li moved into our hostel when his parents entered the refugee camp. This gave him the opportunity to go to the Thai school during the day and attend our English, Bible, and health classes in the evening.

The Thai school changed Pov Li's tribal name to Pak Dee. One Thursday evening at our devotions he argued vigorously against Christianity. The following Saturday he was sitting in my study trying to read the Bible. A Thai soldier came to my study wishing to be baptized. As I talked with him and explained baptism, Pak Dee spoke up. To my surprise he said, "I want to be baptized, too." So Private Lantom and Pak Dee were baptized in the beautiful Khwang River. More of this story in the next case history.

Sunday morning I took my medical bag with me to Paklang Camp. After church I went over to Xai Suav's home.

The dying man said, "Doctor, I do not need the shot today. I feel no more pain. I want you to sit by me and read to me about the new Home I will be entering when I die. Everyone wonders why I have lived so long. I have prayed that God would keep me alive until Pov Li (Pak Dee) became a Christian. Now that he follows God, I know that he can head my family on the right path."

Exhausted, he stopped talking. The family was all gathered around as I read the description of heaven in the last two chapters of Revelation. As he took his final breaths, his facial expression became peacefully radiant. With his last breath he raised one finger and was gone.

They did not scream or curse as is usual among the White Hmong when someone dies. His widow addressed the nine children. "Your father has left his cancer behind. If we are faithful to Jesus, we will meet him in heaven."

⌖ ⌖ ⌖

The fall months of 1972 were disastrous for the malaria situation. The weather was unseasonably warm so the *anopheles* mosquitoes that carry malaria did not die out. Consequently, our hospital was overflowing with malaria cases. Alarmingly most of the cases proved resistant to the newer antimalarial drugs. We had to resort to old-fashioned quinine dripped into the veins.

Falciparum or malignant malaria produced delirium and restlessness. We usually started our malaria patients on mats on the floor. When the high fever and disorientation subsided, the patient could be promoted to a bed.

Private Lantom was one such patient. A powerfully built young man from Bangkok, we had difficulty subduing him enough to put in an IV. The morning after his admission he was rational but deeply depressed.

"Why don't you just let me die, Doctor?" he said. "Spend your time and energy on patients who want to recover. I am twenty-two-years-old and have seen nothing in life that makes me want to keep living."

I replied, "I am twice your age and enjoying a life full of meaning and purpose."

Surang overheard the conversation and limped over to the bedside with a small New Testament. "If you read this book you will understand what the doctor is talking about," she said. "This book has changed my life and brought me much joy." Hesitantly the soldier accepted the book.

The following morning on my hospital rounds I was delighted to see Private Lantom sitting up in his bed smiling. "If this book is true," he exclaimed, "This is what I have been looking for!"

Saturday morning was my half-day of catching up on correspondence and working on my teaching and preaching outlines. I got up early to do my hospital rounds. Private Lantom had recovered so well that I told him he would be dismissed from the hospital the following day.

We seldom had electricity in the mornings, so my desk was next to the window where I could utilize daylight to do the paperwork. Our tall jackfruit tree shaded the desk from direct sunlight.

Suddenly a dark shadow stole my daylight. I had locked the study door, but Private Lantom was standing at the window. A wave of anger and frustration swept over me.

"I have already seen you in the hospital today," I berated him. "You are not dismissed yet. If you have additional concerns, you should tell the nurse and she can contact me. I am very busy now, so you need to go back to the hospital."

Pvt. Lantom was apologetic. "I beg your forgiveness for disturbing you, Doctor," he began. "When I am discharged tomorrow, I will be sent back into the jungle to fight. I have read through the New Testament three times and want to follow Jesus. I was going to ask you to baptize me today."

I felt embarrassed about my outburst. I opened the door and invited him in. With further teaching and questioning, I felt confident that he was ready for baptism.

Pak Dee asked if he could also be baptized. Astonished I asked him, "Just Thursday you were arguing against Christianity. Now, why do you want to be baptized?"

"The change in my parents' lives and your explanation of God's Word have convinced me," he replied.

After further questions and discussion, accompanied by Dorothy and some of the hostel kids, we walked down to the river for the baptism. As they came out of the water, the soldier from Bangkok hugged the tribal refugee boy. "Now we are brothers!" declared the soldier.

We learned later about his life before coming to the hospital. Private Lantom was His Royal Highness Prince Lantom Seniwong na Ayuthya. After graduating from a prestigious university in Bangkok, he received a position in a government ministry. Corruption in that department led to disillusionment and deep depression. He planned to commit suicide but knew that this would bring grief and shame to the Royal family.

He decided to meet his death in a way that would bring honor to the family. He resigned his government position and enlisted as a volunteer for frontline combat duty on the frontier, intending to stand up in front of enemy fire. Instead of a Communist bullet, he was brought down by a mosquito. Instead of dying on a battlefield, he died to his old life and was buried with Christ in baptism.

Socially and culturally few people could be further apart than a university-educated royal prince and a semi-literate tribal refugee boy. Only in Jesus could they be declared "brothers."

Nearly two years later as we were waiting in the Bangkok Airport for our flight back to the United States, Prince Lantom came to send us off. He was radiant in his joy as he shared the opportunities he had to share his faith with the Royal family.

Twenty-three years after leaving Thailand, we returned for a visit. In Chiang Mai, we saw Pak Dee now a full-time preacher of the gospel. We visited in his home and renewed our friendship with his mother, Xai Suav's widow.

Study Questions

1. A potential epidemic of intestinal anthrax was averted by the quick response by the medical staff and district authorities. Because of his efforts, Garland made a significant contribution to medical science in the prevention of a deadly epidemic. He concludes this story with a powerful statement. What is the statement?
2. Read 1 Corinthians 10:31. Garland could have proudly taken all the credit for his actions. Instead he chose to

give all the glory to God. Isn't it amazing what God puts into the minds of man? To whom are we to give the credit for the successful surgeries?

3. Read Isaiah 43:7. God formed and made each one of us. What does this verse say about why we were created?

4. Read Jeremiah 9:23-24. The Lord clearly tells us what to do when we are tempted to brag about something or be praised for something we did or have. The verse says "let him who glories glory in this…" What is it?

5. While Garland and Dorothy were driving their children home from school through darkened hills, they were flagged down by men in combat gear. As Garland stumbled through the dark towards the car to be repaired, what did he do?

6. Read Psalm 77:14. When you are in a frightening or dangerous situation, remember the author of this Psalm and what he did to find strength. What came to his mind to calm him?

7. It is okay to say to God, "Please, God, I know you have delivered miracles in the past, and I'm asking for you to send one right now." Is there somewhere in your life that you need a miracle …. quickly? Was Garland's prayer for a "mechanical miracle" answered?

8. The stories of Pak Dee and Private Lantom were intertwined because of their new found desires to be baptized and follow Jesus. For Private Lantom, his eyes were opened by reading the New Testament. What was it for Pak Dee that made him want to be baptized?

9. The Message Bible gives a wonderful paraphrase of Philippians 2:14-16: "Do everything readily and cheerfully—no bickering, no second-guessing allowed! Go out into the world uncorrupted, a breath of fresh air in this squalid and polluted society. Provide people with a glimpse of good living and of the living God. Carry the light-giving Message into the night so I'll have good cause to be proud of you on the day that Christ returns." How can you live your life as a breath of fresh air to those around you?

Chapter 16

Divine Appointments & Changed Lives

In our ministry in Thailand, we saw God at work doing what seemed impossible. This chapter will give five case studies of lives transformed by the power of Christ:

- The Sorcerer--becomes a clinic chaplain
- The Bear Feeder--learns to feed the flock of God
- The Outlaw--retraces his path of cattle rustling, robbing, and murdering to spread the Good News
- The Seeker--a lifelong search for God and salvation is rewarded by an unwelcome visitor
- The Urchin--an illiterate tribal kid with an attitude becomes a teacher and pastor.

The Sorcerer

Every culture has its practitioners of black arts--be they the wizards and witches of Europe, the witch doctors of Africa, the shamans of Siberia and Tibet, or the voodoo priests of Haiti. Among the many tribes of Thailand, each one had its conjurers or spirit doctors.

In 1953 while living in Chiangkham, we enjoyed a delightful visit from Edgar and Mable Nichols. Uncle Edgar was my mother's brother. They had worked with my parents among the Tibetan people and had escaped the Communist takeover by a harrowing trip over the Himalayas into the part of India then known as Assam. There they found a ready ministry among the Khasi tribal Christians who had studied their way out of denominationalism. My sister Marguerite Fairbrother and her husband Archie joined them and spent seventeen years among the Khasis.

The Nicholses were on their way back to the United States. Uncle Edgar expressed a desire to visit the hill tribes. Since he used to ride horses, we borrowed a couple of horses and climbed up to a Hmong village. As yet I could not speak either of the Hmong dialects and only a smattering of Northern Thai.

We carried a wind-up phonograph and some gospel recordings in the Hmong language. We also had some pictorial charts illustrating the plan of salvation. I stumbled through an evangelistic message in the northern Thai dialect, but the tribesmen only appeared baffled.

Soon a man who partially understood my message joined the crowd around the fire. He was a northern Thai from the Chiangkham plain. He explained to me that he was selling charms and amulets to the tribespeople.

The message of Jesus and His power over demons fascinated this man, JunTa. While Uncle Ed silently prayed, I stumbled through the story of Jesus. JunTa asked if he could visit me in Chiangkham to learn more about the power of Pra Yesu. This gentle sad-faced man appeared to have a genuine spiritual hunger.

How disappointed Mel Byers and I were when JunTa came to visit us. Like Simon the sorcerer in Acts 8:9-13, his main motive appeared to be material profit from marketing the power of Jesus. We firmly told him that salvation was not for sale.

In spite of the rebuke, JunTa kept coming back and we watched his attitude change to the earnest seeking of a troubled soul. He developed a hunger and thirst for righteousness exemplified in Pra Yesu.

The day came when JunTa confessed his faith in Pra Yesu and Mel Byers baptized him. As a new believer, he soon led his best friend to Christ.

JunTa became an avid student of the Bible. One day he and his friend received a summons to appear before the local magistrate. His conversion to Christ had created a furor in the community.

At first apprehensive, JunTa found his fears calmed by reading Matthew 10:19-20. In this passage Christ assured His followers that the Holy Spirit will give them the words to say when they appeared before rulers.

At the trial the angry magistrate opened the proceedings: "You are charged, Nai [Mr.] JunTa, not only with leaving our Buddhist tradition and adopting the foreigners' religion, but stirring up controversy by misleading your best friend to follow you. You are disturbing the township by your teaching."

JunTa replied: "Your Honor, I am not alone on trial today. His Majesty King Mongkut is also on trial for inviting the American missionaries into Thailand to build schools and hospitals. The Thai Parliament is on trial for drafting laws granting religious freedom to all citizens of the kingdom. Besides, your Honor, Pra Yesu was not an American or

European. He lived and taught in our own continent of Asia. One does not need to cross any sea to reach the land where He ministered."

"Case dismissed," declared the magistrate.

As we prepared to move to Pua, Mel Byers continued to mentor JunTa. The former sorcerer prayed for opportunities to expand his ministry.

Dorothy Uhlig, a highly-trained missionary, had come to Thailand a few months before our arrival in 1951. Besides being a registered nurse, she was trained in midwifery, Bible, and linguistics. Like us, she had originally planned to go to Tibet. She started out ministering to the leprosy villages but soon opened a clinic in Chiangkham. Mel Byers and Imogene Williams, both trained in missionary medicine, assisted her. They needed a clinic evangelist fluent in the local dialects and passionate for Jesus.

When offered the position, JunTa expressed delight and served ably as the clinic evangelist for nearly forty years. Dorothy Uhlig completed sixty-two years of dedicated service when she went to be with the Lord in June 2013.

The Bear Feeder

Trekking up to the Frost Pocket required a steep ascent and descent over "Unnecessary Mountain," our nickname for PhuWae. The climb required a nearly vertical ascent to the Lua village of Sakat, famous for its pickled tea leaves or *mieng*. Tea bushes grew throughout the village, and the leaves were harvested at a certain stage. These were pickled in brine and wadded around garlic to make a refreshing, stimulating chew.

Leaving Sakat the trail followed a steep treeless ridge where the hot sun beat down while we struggled through the sharp blades of *kha* or roofing grass. Exposed skin on the neck and arms could be marked with slashes like paper cuts.

A rain forest covered the summit, a welcome relief from the hot ridge. But it had its own vexations. Voracious leeches swarmed on the leaves along the trail ready to latch onto the unwary traveler.

We tucked our pant legs into our boots and slathered odoriferous World War II insect repellent on our clothing and exposed skin. The native couriers accompanying me made no such precautions. They smoked home-made cigars that had a repellent effect. If they touched an attached leech with the burning end of the cigar, the leech would drop off immediately.

Descending from the rain forest we encountered a hot, scrubby area where we stopped to attend to our leech bites. When biting, the leech injects two kinds of chemicals into the victim. It starts with a local anesthetic so the victim does not feel the bite. An anti-coagulant follows so the blood will flow freely.

Serious blood loss can follow. My companions gathered the leaves of a tall weed, called *Eupatorium odoratum,* which grew by the trail. They crushed the leaves into a poultice. Applied to the wound the poultice stopped the bleeding almost immediately. (Dr. Ralph Cozort, visiting Professor of Pharmacology at Chiang Mai Medical College, later found that *Eupatorium* contains a powerful clotting agent.)

Near the base of "Unnecessary Mountain," we came to a cornfield with abundant ripening ears. As we arrived, we met a sturdy young Hmong man leaving the field with a basket of newly picked ears.

"Where are you taking the corn?" I asked. With an embarrassed laugh, he replied, "To feed the bear. A bear has a den among the boulders yonder. By taking the food near its den, I am hoping it will leave my cornfield alone."

"I never heard of bribing a bear," I said laughing. He joined me in laughter as he lay down his basket.

"I can deliver the food later. Come to the field hut and talk with me," he urged. At the side of the field stood a crude hut built of rough-hewn planks, bamboo poles, and a grass roof. A family member stayed in the hut during harvest to ward off marauding animals. One side was completely open.

We sat down in the shelter. He told me his name was Tswv Sab and that he was the son of the chieftain that Mel Byers and I had visited a few years earlier. He displayed a thirst for all kinds of knowledge. When I mentioned that we had the Blue Hmong primer that would help him learn to read and write his own language, he became quite excited. "When harvest is over, may I come to your house and learn to read?" he inquired. I assured him he would be welcome.

As we proceeded to the Frost Pocket, little did I foresee how his life would become entwined with ours. In our newsletters, Tswv Sab would be referred to as "Lao Jur," as he was called by those outside the tribe.

After corn harvest, Tswv Sab showed up at our home with his bedroll, pencils, and notepaper. We fed him at our table and spent as much time as possible teaching him from the primer and sharing the life of Jesus with him.

He could only stay one week, but in that week he had mastered the first primer. He was thrilled that the Bible was being translated into the Hmong language and urged us to hurry up and finish it.

As Tswv Sab prepared to leave, I asked him if anything about the life and teachings of Yexu impressed him or raised questions. He replied that the teachings about Yexu did not impress as much as the fact that my wife and I sat at the table together and were friends.

In pre-Christian Hmong culture, a man kidnapped a woman for his bride, followed by haggling with the bride's parents over the bride price. The wife then had the status of a work animal and was subjected to beatings and verbal abuse. At meals men and boys were served first. When the men were through eating, the women and girls ate the leftovers. Many of the men became opium addicts in their thirties and forties, leaving the women to do most of the house and field work.

We continued to have numerous contacts with Tswv Sab and eventually rejoiced when he confessed his faith and was baptized. Impetuous and somewhat unstable he reminded us of Simon Peter's early years as a disciple. For every step backward, he appeared to take two steps forward. Soon the growing Hmong church viewed him as a leader.

Communist terrorists from across the border in Laos began to harass the Hmong villages including Kang Haw in the Frost Pocket. Tribespeople, who chose to be loyal to the Thai government, were driven to the valley below from their mountain villages.

The Thai government resettled them in a refugee camp at Paklang just east of Pua. These refugees included Blue Hmong,

White Hmong, Lua, and Mienh. Believers among the refugees built a chapel with plank benches and vertical palm slats under a grass roof. Services began mid-morning and continued to mid-afternoon.

Tswv Sab became quite an effective elder. Three of his children moved to our hostel and became outspoken Christians. His older daughter, Sukanya, became like a daughter to us. We all experienced deep grief when she developed bone cancer and had to have her leg amputated. During her hospitalization in Chiang Mai, she led a medical student and some nurses to the Lord.

When we left Thailand, their entire family was flourishing spiritually.

The Outlaw

Don and Roberta Byers began a ministry with the Khmu tribe in the village of Nam Mong on the Yao River. A few miles downstream was the Thai-Lu village of Ban Haan, the lair of the brigand, Saeng Pua.

Saeng Pua was known as a robber, murderer, and rustler of water buffalo and other cattle. He had wives and children scattered in several villages. When stealing cattle, he would conceal them in the remote, isolated village of Ban Pong Lom ("Mud Hole Village").

The eight families in this village were grudging protectors of Saeng Pua's booty. They feared his reprisals if they did not cooperate. On the other hand, they were fearful of government penalties should the concealed animals be discovered.

The Khmu response to the gospel alarmed Saeng Pua. Feeling that a growing acceptance of the gospel threatened his livelihood, he launched a personal counterattack.

As Don Byers preached to the villagers, Saeng Pua tried to disrupt the services with mocking. He jeered when Don mispronounced a word. He challenged the crowd, "Are you going to allow these Americans to capture you with their strange doctrines? They will make you slaves to fight against the Russians."

One day I had the opportunity to preach in Nam Mong. As usual Saeng Pua heckled me as the speaker and disrupted the service.

I preached about God's forgiveness--coming to Christ in repentant obedience could wipe our slate clean from past sin. He challenged me, "Do you know who I am?"

"Yes. I know who you are," I replied.

He began recounting details of his criminal past. "Do you mean that God can forgive all of that?"

"Yes, He can and He will," I replied, "if you come to Him in penitent faith."

His heckling stopped. He stood silently attentive while I completed my message.

Soon afterward, we heard the thrilling news of Saeng Pua's confession of faith and baptism. He wanted to make changes to atone for his past crimes.

Speaking with Don, he said, "I cannot restore life to those I murdered. I cannot return everything I stole. What can I do about the wives and children I have in other villages?"

Saeng Pua decided to return to live with his first wife and make provision for the other women and children. His gang dissolved and at least one of them became a Christian. He decided he would retrace his steps to the villages he had plundered while apologizing and sharing the good news of his new life in Christ.

He became a leader in the new church at his village of Ben Haan. He never learned to read, but insisted that his children receive schooling. It was a joy to him to sit on the veranda of his house while his sons read the Bible to him. When we left Thailand he was well respected in the Christian community.

On our return visit to Thailand in 1997, we learned that he had remained faithful to the end of his life. The Ban Haan church was still flourishing.

One of his sons is an evangelist. He visited with us telling of his recent trip to Communist China where he was able to lead hundreds of the Thai-Lu to Christ.

Virgilio and Esther de los Santos, veteran missionaries from the Philippines continue to guide and encourage the Ban Haan church.

The Seeker

Tip was born to a poor family in Lampang, the second largest city in Northern Thailand famed for its Buddhist temples and highly educated monks. His parents discouraged him from becoming a monk but were diligent in offering cooked rice with bamboo sprouts to the yellow-robed monks who passed by their door every morning.

Tip had a thirst for knowledge, but his parents did not allow him to go to school, saying they could not afford the required uniforms. He went to the temple frequently with his parents, sitting cross-legged on the cool pavement with his palms pressed together in the *wai* posture of prayer. The monks chanted scriptures in the Pali dialect. The hearers did not understand the words but hoped to gain merit in the quest to escape the misery of reincarnation.

The young man carried burning questions to the abbot. How was this world formed? Is there a supreme being? Where can we find joy? How can one be cleansed from sin?

The answers did not satisfy him. "It is not ours to know the origins or creator. Life is suffering. One should not seek joy. Do good deeds to atone for your sins. If your good deeds outweigh your bad, you will be reincarnated to a better life."

Frustrated, Tip shook his head. "Is there anyone who might have more answers?" he asked.

"Your questions are impertinent," replied the abbot. "A holy hermit lives in a cave in the mountains above Phayao Lake. He does nothing but meditate on the great teachings."

Tip trekked northeast to the mountains overlooking Phayao Lake. With anticipation he climbed the trail to the hermit's cave. Expecting to find a serene holy man, he was shocked to find a cranky old man who berated him for looking for answers beyond what the abbot had taught him.

"You will not find any different answers in our country," the hermit told him. "However, if you are determined to keep looking, consider the temples of Mandalay where the priests have reached the summits of learning from the scriptures of the Lord Buddha."

Weeks of walking through northwestern Thailand and Burma finally brought him to the golden spires of Mandalay. He could speak no Burmese, but the Shan people of Burma spoke a dialect of the Thai language. A friendly Shan man guided him to the monks of Mandalay and served as his interpreter though Tip only partially understood his dialect.

The Burmese monks treated the young seeker from Thailand with amused disdain. He was receiving no answers to the yearning of his hungry soul. Disillusioned with Buddhism, Tip returned to Thailand with a prayer from his heart, "God, if there is a god, send me a messenger to bring light to my eyes and peace to my heart."

Scripture assures us, "Seek the LORD your God and you will find him, if you search after him with all your heart and with all your soul" (Deuteronomy 4:29). Jesus adds, "If anyone's will is to do God's will, he will know whether the teaching is from God or whether I am speaking on my own authority" (John 7:17).

Back at Lampang, Tip took up the occupation of an itinerant peddler. Buying cloth and other sundries in Lampang, he would go to distant villages and sell them for a small profit. Near Pua, he met a petite, pretty girl and fell in love. He gave up peddling to settle to life as a rice farmer with his father-in-law.

After the death of the father-in-law, Tip became head of the household. It caused consternation when he refused to pay taxes to support the village *wat* (temple). The village chieftain called a meeting. "If you do not support our *wat*, you must leave the village," he decreed.

Tip decided to reclaim some boggy timbered wetlands and start a new village--Ban Pong Lom. Four other families helped form Mudhole Village. Disillusioned with Buddhism he decided to wait for answers to his questions. Passing middle age, Tip was universally referred to as Uncle Tip.

Sitting on his veranda one afternoon, Uncle Tip saw an unwelcome sight. Saeng Pua, the outlaw, had entered the village and was approaching. As he neared the house, Uncle Tip addressed him, "What mischief are you up to now?"

"No mischief this time. I have come in love. I have met God and He has given me a new heart. I want to apologize for all the grief I have caused you."

"Come up here and sit by me," Uncle Tip demanded, "This sounds like what I have been searching for these many years."

Saeng Pua explained how he had met Christ. "Let me go get Grandfather Gaao from Pua. He can read God's Book and explain 'how to enter through Pra Yesu.'"

Grandpa Gaao was a rice farmer who was one of the first to be baptized in Pua. He loved to travel from village to village preaching Christ. Saeng Pua and Grandpa Gaao returned to Ban Pong Lom and taught for several days. All of the adults in the village believed and were baptized.

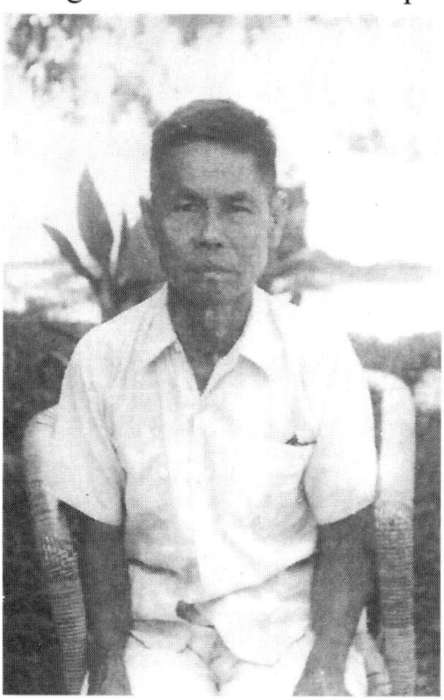

Grandpa Gaao

A few days later we were thrilled to visit the first church in the district to be formed before they had met a foreign missionary.

The Strong-willed Child

On one of my visits to Kang Haw in the Frost Pocket, I taught from a pictorial chart of the life of Christ. Unbathed children of all ages crowded around me as I struggled to teach by the light of a kerosene pressure lantern. We met in the home of the village headman. They called him the honorific Lao Ta. I do not remember his actual name.

Lao Ta was progressive in his views. He desired economic and educational progress for his tribe. Pointing out a group of boys in the eight to ten-year-old range, he said, "My son and nephews want to go to school. If we sent them to Pua, could they live with you?"

I explained to him that we did not have a sleeping room in the house we lived in, but we would try to make room for them at the beginning of the following dry season. He introduced three shy boys: Teng (Teem), his son, Lee (Li), his nephew, and Ya (Yag), son of a cousin.

To our dismay, on an August afternoon in the height of the rainy season Lao Ta and his brother showed up with the three wet, muddy urchins. They had just struggled across the flooded Pua River.

We faced an urgent list of to-do's:

- Give them thin Thai bath towels to wrap in while we laundered their muddy clothes.

- Lay mats on the end of the porch and hang privacy curtains.
- Send their fathers to the market to buy school uniforms.
- Cut off their "ponytails" because this would make them a laughing-stock to the Thai people and would prevent their admission to a Thai school.
- Remove the silver rings from their necks and scrub off the black tarnish in the process of giving what might have been their first complete baths.
- Cook a hot, nourishing meal.
- Find enough cotton blankets for the night.

The following day began another long list of responsibilities:

- Begin teaching them rudimentary Thai so they could begin school.
- Enroll them in the local school.
- Teach them basic table manners and the use of utensils.
- Arrange for the parents to provide rice. We would help with vegetables and meat.
- Order Kapok mattresses.
- Build a partition for their bedroom.

The Thai teachers renamed the boys with Thai names. Nine-year-old Li became Chalee. Ten-year-old Teng became Tengtrairat, shortened to the original Teng. Ya, the other ten-year-old, became Banya. Banya, being strong-willed, resisted obeying orders. His temper tantrums presented a real challenge.

One day he became angry with Dorothy. He climbed to the top of our tallest tree. From the treetop, he cursed Dorothy. "I will stay here until I die," he threatened, "or until that old woman dies."

Dorothy was firm about assigning duties: cooking, laundry, drawing water from the well, and homework. On Thursday evenings, we had a trilingual Bible study and also taught them to sing hymns. They became like brothers to Geoffrey and Corinne.

We watched the transforming power of the gospel and a loving home affect their lives. The older boys became honor students covering two academic years each year until they caught up with their age group. Chalee did not have scholarly inclinations and quit school after one year, returning to farming with his parents. He found the ability to read and speak Thai quite advantageous. As far as we know, he never became a Christian.

Teng and Banya became excited about the life and message of Jesus. Their baptism brought us great joy. We saw a remarkable transformation in Banya's life and attitude. No more tantrums. No more stubborn rebellion.

Teng's parents came to the Lord. His mother became a radiant outgoing Christian, prominent in the life of the Paklang Church. We felt that Teng and his father Lao Ta failed to reach their spiritual potential. Teng graduated from high school with honors and went on to a career of teaching.

After graduation, Banya went to a Bible training school, then on to agricultural college. Fellow students heckled him for his faith. He spent a lot of time in a field hut among the experimental test plots guarding the precious crops from marauding animals.

In his research project he raised egg-laying *coturnix* quails. Quail eggs are a popular menu item in Asian restaurants.

After completing agricultural college, he accepted a teaching position as an agriculture instructor in Wang Pa High School in Nan Province. He built a home for his family with a wing used as a hostel for offering Bible training to tribal youth.

Banya preached and taught in many tribal churches. He served as peacemaker and mediator in many church disputes. We received news in June 2013 that the Paklang Church called Banya as their preaching minister.

Study Questions

This chapter tells five case studies of lives transformed by the power of Christ.

The Sorcerer

1. JunTa seemed to be fascinated when hearing about Jesus and his power over demons. Ed was praying as Garland shared the Gospel message. What do you think Ed was praying? If so, were his prayers answered?

2. Read Titus 3:3-7. How do these verses relate to the story of JunTa? By God's mercy and grace, JunTa was reborn and renewed into one now with the hope of eternal life. If there is someone you know who needs to hear the Good News of Jesus, but you are not sure what to say, read Matthew 10:19-20 as JunTa did. These are the

verses that calmed his fears when he had to explain his faith.

The Bear Feeder

3. While making the treacherous journey down the mountain, Garland's group just happened to run into a young Hmong man, Tswv Sab. How has a chance encounter, i.e. being at the right place at the right time, somehow changed your life forever?

4. Read Proverbs 16:9. Was anyone in Garland's group intentionally looking for someone with whom they could share the Gospel on that grueling trip? Even when we are not intentional, God is! He is making heavenly assignments and connections all the time, so we need to pay attention when He nudges us to speak to someone in our path.

5. A divine appointment is when God brings someone across your path on purpose either for you to spiritually encourage or for you to be encouraged. Read Acts 8:26-35. It seemed God was leading Philip into the middle of nowhere, but on the road, who did he encounter? What happened at this divine appointment?

The Outlaw

6. Saeng Pua had a history as a pretty bad man, wouldn't you say? His list of sins was long and included robbery, murder, theft, and adultery. When he recounted details of his past, what question did he ask? What was Garland's

answer? Why would that be difficult to accept if you had made bad choices in your past?

7. Read Romans 3:23-24. How many of us have sinned and fallen short of the glory of God? Again, do you think "all" really means ALL? What are your thoughts on this statement: It is impossible to outsin the grace of God.

8. When someone as sinful as Saeng Pua (or as sinful as you and me) accepts Jesus as Savior and starts a new life in Christ, would that be considered a miracle?

The Seeker

9. Read 1 John 1:7-9. What is the first step toward receiving forgiveness of past sins?

The Urchin – Strong Willed Child

10. Garland and Dorothy watched the transforming power of the gospel and a loving home affected the lives of three young boys. Read Deuteronomy 6:6-9. What does the Bible teach us about raising children to know the Lord?

11. If you have raised children to know and love Jesus, are there other children whom you can reach for Christ? What are some ideas of connecting with children in families where they do not attend church or teach about Jesus in their homes?

Part Three

Transition in Ministry

Chapter 17

Provision for Departure

Events moved toward a close in our term in Pua. Being on call 24/7 with no vacations and no time for continuing medical education kept me battling through a fog of fatigue. Geoffrey and Corinne were in their final years of high school and would be considering college choices. Grace Eileen needed additional physical therapy and special education as well as seizure control. Managing accounts and correspondence, overseeing the daily needs of more than twenty tribal youngsters, participating in outreach to refugees and serving as a hostess to overnight guests on a nearly daily basis pushed Dorothy to the brink of total exhaustion.

We desperately missed our parents and siblings after the years apart. Our nephews and nieces did not remember us. We needed to return to the United States--but how? We had no financial reserves. The churches and individuals who had faithfully supported us from the beginning continued their support. However, in those days most church budgets did not provide repatriation and retirement funds for missionaries. Nevertheless experience had taught us that where God leads, he provides.

A business trip took me to Chiangkam where we had started our mission life. The Mel Byers family and Dorothy Uhlig still lived and worked there. Previously a trip on foot required nearly a week. Now the military situation had caused the Thai government to build an all-weather road that cut travel time to less than a day. It was exciting to drive on this new strip of asphalt as it cut through the hills where we had once taught, sweaty and caked with dust.

On this bright, beautiful, and relatively cool day high speeds were not possible with chickens, humped oxen, water buffalo, and children trying out the new thoroughfare. Roaming dogs and plodding peasants were oblivious to the perils of motor traffic. As I drove up a rather steep hill and neared the crest, I received a strong impulse, "STOP!" I heard no audible voice, but I slowed to a crawl. Reaching the summit, I could see the road ahead. Just below the hilltop a huge bull buffalo stood in my lane of the road. Had I not stopped in time the "Blue Bus" and probably its driver would have been demolished. The buffalo would have been disabled and provided a village feast.

But what about the message to stop? Was it ESP or pure coincidence? I believe it was a message from a loving heavenly Father to protect His servant for further service.

What about the future of the hostel? We rejoiced that Imogene Williams would be taking charge after we left. The tribal youngsters were overflowing the space. What would it cost to build a boys' dorm? Also, a new dormitory for girls and a home for Imogene Williams would need to be constructed. Priority would be the boys' dorm. We already had twelve boys in senior high school.

I figured the cost for lumber and labor including plumbing and electricity and it was considerably beyond our means. Would it be worthwhile given the unstable condition of our border province? We earnestly prayed for guidance.

We had a surprise visit from Dr. Geoffrey Atkinson who served with the British forces in the Vietnam War. As a Christian, Dr. Atkinson was keenly interested in our mission work. A few weeks after his visit we received a letter from him including a check large enough to cover the cost of the boys' dormitory. We accepted this as a go-ahead order to proceed with building.

In subsequent months, we saw the completion of Imogene's home and the girl's dormitory. It was great to have Imogene and her delightful adopted daughter Tina as next-door neighbors.

What is the greatest hardship about leaving the mission field? Saying goodbye to those who have become your new family is hard. Sorting and packing brought excruciating decisions since we had to leave behind most of our possessions. Collecting travel documents, planning itineraries, purchasing tickets all create multiple headaches. For me as an incurable Type A personality, being polite to well-wishers who "waste my time" was a tribulation. For years I had tried to treat my interruptions as opportunities, but that usually created inner turmoil. Thank God, Dorothy is much more laid back and not a slave to the clock.

One morning in the flurry of sorting and packing, a village farmer of the Lu tribe interrupted my schedule. I did not recognize him, but he seemed to know me. I smiled through gritted teeth while he made small talk. My brain was screaming, "Get to the point! I don't have all day!"

Finally, he got to the point. "Your sermon got through to me. I am ready to follow."

"What sermon? When?" I inquired.

"Sixteen years ago you came to our village and told us about Pra Yesu [Jesus], Son of the Creator, who has power over demons. I'm tired of fighting demons and ready to follow Pra Yesu."

Being close to our departure, I could not go with him back to his village. The man who had gone with me on the previous trip accompanied him to his village. He witnessed to others, seeking to persuade them to join him in being baptized.

Had we not experienced years of provision from the hands of Jehovah Jireh (God Who Provides) we might have been in major anxiety at the financial cliff towering ahead. We had an invitation to conduct a speaking itinerary in Australia and New Zealand. High school graduations and college experiences loomed for our two older children. Rehabilitation and special education lay ahead for Grace Eileen.

Since we had never used a credit card and had no credit rating, we wondered how we could get a house and a car when we arrived in the States. How would the Great Provider meet these needs? The answer came from Thunder Bay, Ontario.

Miss Mattie Babcock was a distant cousin of my father who spent many years as a school teacher in Thunder Bay. Through my Dad, she had followed our work on the mission field. We had never been to Thunder Bay and had never met her. On a teacher's salary, she must have lived quite frugally for the bequest she left us after her death enabled us to cover all the looming expenses.

Study Questions

1. While traveling to Chiangkam, Garland received a strong impulse to stop the car which in turn, prevented a likely fatal accident. How did he explain the inaudible voice he "heard?"

2. Read Proverbs 3:5. There was no way the much-needed boys' dorm could be built with the lack of money at that time, and the area was unstable as well. Rather than leaning on their own understanding, what did Garland and Dorothy do?

3. Dr. Atkinson made a surprise visit to see what was happening with the ongoing mission work, then followed up shortly after with a large check to build the dormitory. Would you call this a coincidence or a miracle?

4. Read 2 Corinthians 9:8-11. How do these verses give encouragement when there is a need for guidance and provision?

5. An answer to prayers for provision for the moving expenses came from an unlikely person halfway around the world. Though family, the Bares had never met their distant cousin. God used a stranger's generosity to provide for the needs of his servants. Does God orchestrate everything, like death at just the time Miss Babcock's gift would help the Bares the most?

6. Read Philippians 4:10-19. The Apostle Paul is thanking those who provided for his needs as he dedicated his life to spreading the Good News of Jesus. In verse 17, Paul said it wasn't that he desired those gifts. What did he desire? What did he mean by having "credit to your account?"

7. Do you know about the missionary or mission organizations your church supports with regular financial gifts? Maybe you know of a young person or couple who have been called to do mission work abroad, in your community, or perhaps on a college campus. To offer support to someone you know or do as Miss Babcock did, support someone you have never met is to not just bless them, but to receive God's blessings on you. What are some ideas on how you can support mission work with your money and your prayers?

Chapter 18

Transitional Trauma & Reflections on Ministry

The thought of leaving our beloved Thailand with no definite prospect of returning overwhelmed us. Behind us were the years of language study and adaptation to primitive living conditions.

We came to Thailand determined to "put the old American to death" clearing the slate for adapting to the mindset and culture of the people to whom we had been called. Living without electricity, all-weather roads, and grocery stores felt more like a prolonged camping adventure than a period of privation.

We yearned for communication with our loved ones in the United States. Mail took two to three weeks. Transcontinental telephone and jet travel were not available. We tried to get off a monthly prayer letter to our support base.

With prayerful advice from our fellow workers, we had moved to Pua as our base of operations in 1954. We arrived, not by invitation of the people, but by commission of our Commander. As the first Americans to live in the district, we encountered curiosity by all, hostility by some, and friendliness from few.

With the birth of baby Geoffrey, Dorothy found rapport with the young mothers of the village. Parents restricted newly weaned babies to a diet of rice and salt, leaving them with severe vitamin deficiency.

Vitamin A deficiency causes thick scarring of the cornea and blindness. Papayas, a rich source of vitamin A, grew in abundance, but the people in our district only used it as food for pigs. Dorothy started little Geoff on ripe papayas when he began to eat cereal and fruit.

"Look, she's feeding him pig food!" exclaimed the astonished villagers. Observing how the white baby thrived broke down their resistance. Soon papayas became baby food and we saw no more blind toddlers. The citrus groves started spreading in our district and vitamin A deficiency became a thing of the past among youngsters.

In 1956 a daughter Lois Corinne joined our family and Dorothy became primarily a stay-at-home mom. She started a Bible study class for the children of Pua using flannel graph as a teaching aid. Attendance increased week-by-week as they enthusiastically sang the new songs about Jesus.

The counterattack came swiftly. A speaker was brought in from a famous *wat* (temple) in Lampang. He held a "revival" in the Pua temple using a gas-powered generator to broadcast his sermons audibly all over the town. We heard him warn the townsfolk. "Keep your children away from the American missionaries. Buddhism is our national Thai religion and we must stay faithful to it." To our disappointment, the children stopped coming.

Years later a Christian Thai lady living in Chicago visited us. "I started my journey of faith in the children's services in Pua many years ago," she stated. Another reminder that the Good News seed is not sown in vain.

We focused on evangelism among the Hmong, especially the Blue Hmong sub-tribe. This would involve many steps. Locating their villages by climbing the mountain to their altitude level.

- Finding an informant to help learn their language.
- Analyzing the consonants, vowels, and tones.
- Developing a written language.
- Developing primers in their language.
- Beginning Bible translation.

The missionaries of the Overseas Missionary Fellowship (OMF) did a good deal of this groundwork. We were grateful for their partnership.

Mel Byers and I made the first exploratory trip to the Hmong of Nan Province in 1953. We climbed up to the Frost Pocket, an area northeast of Pua where a bowl-shaped depression surrounded by higher peaks traps cold air. It is one of the few spots in Thailand where frost and freezing temperatures occur in winter.

We stayed in the home of the tribal chief. He spoke the northern Thai dialect quite fluently which was helpful since I was not able to speak Hmong yet. He was full of questions:

- "Where are you from?"
- "How far away is that?"
- Why did you come?"

We explained that when the sun set over his mountains, it was rising in our homeland and that his sunrise coincided with our sunset. We came because God the Creator had delivered us from the power of demons and forgave our sins by sending His Son Yesu to die as an atoning sacrifice. Yesu had risen from the dead and now lives. He has commanded us to share the good news with our brothers and sisters around the world.

"What you tell us must be very important. Why else would you young men leave your parents and come so far? When you learn our language and teach us clearly we may all believe and follow Yesu." Sadly the old chief died before anyone could return with the Good News.

The chief and his village, Kang Haw, were quite progressive and had sent three youths down to Pua to attend the Thai school. These three adolescents were our first informants. Chai Yi was the most helpful. Chai Yi was a quiet solemn youth. I never heard him laugh. However, as he tutored me, he opened his heart to the joyful message of Jesus. We were all jubilant on the day he decided to be baptized.

"Should you talk to your parents before your baptism?" I inquired. "No, I don't think it is necessary," he replied. "They will be happy for me." Little did he know what persecution lay ahead.

Coming out of the water, he was smiling. "Before I believed, I was living in a dark cave. Now I am in the sunlight."

Returning to his village, he walked into a storm of fury and consternation. The village elders harangued him day and night. Only his mother stood up for him. Finally, his father said, "We will do whatever the shaman says we must do."

The spirit-doctor told him he must be "unbaptized." They took him down to the stream where the shaman immersed him out of Jesus and back into demon power.

When we heard this news, it devastated us. The first convert in the Hmong tribe had caved in and denied the Lord. We made our preparations for our first furlough with heavy hearts.

Fatigue and discouragement overwhelmed us as we packed for our first furlough. After three years in Pua, our message had been rejected, our love had met coldness, and very few people could be counted as friends. A jolly policeman, the village midwife, and the Sikh proprietor of the noodle shop with his Shan wife were the only ones who expressed a wish for our return from America.

On the other hand, there was the joyful anticipation of introducing Geoffrey and Corinne to their grandparents, aunts, uncles, and cousins.

We also looked forward to reuniting with our classmates, prayer partners, and supporting churches.

We found our second term somewhat more encouraging. Working with a team of translators, we completed the re-translation of the Old Testament from Hebrew to Thai. Learning of my interest in natural history, Dr. William Smalley the local representative of the American Bible Society asked me to develop a multilingual translator's guide to the plants and animals of the Bible.

The Bible Society noted that I had studied Hebrew and asked me to serve on a committee to revise the entire Thai Old Testament. Pioneer missionaries relied in part on the King James Version in preparing the previous translation. Thai and Hebrew languages are linguistically related to the poetic Sanskrit language. Completing the project provided a sense of relief and joy.

As the number of Hmong believers grew, some of them became convicted that they needed to seek an alternative source of livelihood. With opium being their main cash crop, their awakened consciences told them that they should not profit from a substance that enslaves and degrades thousands of people.

The hill behind our house became a test garden for alternative crops that might thrive in a subtropical climate. Corresponding with agriculturalists in Africa, Latin America, and other parts of Asia we received seed from coffee, macadamia, lychee, scuppernong grapes, cherimoyas, and other subtropical fruits and nuts.

Trekking to mountain villages came to a halt when the doctor diagnosed me with viral cardiomyopathy. Limited life expectancy demanded a change in direction. The physician who cared for me through the illness predicted that I had no more than five years to live.

I rejected the recommendation that I assume a restful sedentary lifestyle while waiting for the inevitable demise. As previously recounted all the barriers to medical school had been removed in unexpected ways.

After completing medical school and a year of residency in surgery, our third term centered on the hostel and medical ministries. Dr. Charoen, a skillful surgeon, joined the Pua hospital team in 1972. This relieved me of a lot of hospital pressure and freed up time for teaching and other ministry.

Early in 1974, the believers asked me to help them with the drug addiction rampant among the hill tribes. Opium was readily available as a painkiller.

We set aside a small building in the backyard as our drug rehabilitation clinic. Most of the addicts were on opium, but we also treated heroin and nicotine addiction. I discovered that nicotine may be the most addicting of all drugs. My patients found opium and heroin easier to give up than nicotine.

We used non-addicting medications to relieve the side effects of withdrawal. Most influential were daily Bible study and frequent prayers.

Substance abuse rehabilitation is most effective when accompanied by deep spiritual transformation. Never underestimate the power of the Holy Spirit! I grieve at the specter of our modern entertainment idols bouncing in and out of rehab programs.

The final month in Pua was extremely painful. The number of believers had grown to a few hundred. The Paklang and Baan Han churches were flourishing. About thirty tribal youngsters occupied the hostel and they were excelling scholastically and growing spiritually. Our hearts broke at leaving all of this behind.

At a farewell conference for believers, Jiem Meng was the main speaker coming all the way from Khon Kaen. Thai, Hmong, and Khmu believers united their voices in praise.

After our tearful final service at the Paklang Church, weeping Hmong women clung to our vehicle as though to prevent our departure.

The Thai government concluded that my medical service and our work with the hill tribes people kept them loyal to the Thai government preventing a Communist takeover of Nan Province. I received the Order of the White Elephant by the Thai, the highest honor given to a non-Thai citizen. The Pua district official honored us with a banquet. Following this, the Governor of Nan Province spread another banquet in Nan.

The Princess Mother (mother of Thailand's king) had previously asked me to serve in the Helicopter Flying Doctors program. I went out on a few missions treating patients in villages inaccessible by road, sometimes behind enemy lines. We also evacuated wounded members of the military.

For these reasons, we were informed that His Majesty would bestow a medal. This was presented in Washington, D.C. after our return to the United States. I was gratified that my mother and Dorothy could be present for the presentation.

The servant of Jesus should not seek the honor of man. When this comes unexpectedly, it should be offered up to God with the prayer that it will contribute to the furtherance of the gospel.

Study Questions

1. As plans were underway to return to America, Garland reflected on the many life-changing experiences for both his family and the people in Thailand. Read 2 Corinthians 11. The Apostle Paul gives an extensive list of the hardships he endured while in ministry. Does it sound foolish to you that someone would willingly put themselves in a position to suffer like Paul did?

2. Read Ephesians 4:1-7. Do you think Garland and Dorothy could have lived the life they did in Thailand without knowing that their work was what they are called to do and prepared to do? What kind of "good works" has God called you to do?

3. Dorothy worked with village children teaching them about Jesus only to have the tribal leaders fight and essentially kill her efforts in 1956. Then, years later, a Christian Thai lady from Chicago shared that she had been one of those children. Read 1 Corinthians 15:58. How does this verse give hope to those who give their lives to serving the Lord, yet do not see results for many years?

4. As Garland received numerous honors, he held true to what Scripture teaches. Reread the last paragraph of this chapter and restate it in your own words.

Chapter 19

Return to America

Farewells ended, we flew from Nan to Bangkok. Then began hundreds of miles by train to Malaysia. Crossing by ferry to the island of Penang we arrived in time for Corinne's graduation from Dalat School. As a surprise graduation gift, Geoffrey flew out from Nebraska Christian College. Several of the graduates gave testimonies of their spiritual growth while at the school. Corinne's graduation with honors did not surprise us.

We sailed from Kuala Lumpur on the *SSMalaysia* bound for Singapore and Perth, Australia. They served us an abundance of foods beginning with an optional breakfast in bed followed by sumptuous snacks and gourmet meals as we sailed through the Indonesian Islands. We had not gorged ourselves so shamelessly since we first arrived in the Orient.

Our feasting ended abruptly when we entered the open Indian Ocean. Our ship tossed on the pitching waves like a cork in a flash flood. The seven hundred passengers lost their appetites en masse and the dining room was empty.

The quieting of the waves on Sunday morning gave a pleasant interlude. We celebrated communion in our cabin with an Australian Christian family.

Our ship arrived late in Perth, so we missed a welcoming party from a Church of Christ there. Port authorities found that we had lived in an opium-growing region near the Golden Triangle, so they gave us quite a grilling.

We boarded a plane for Melbourne where I spoke at a Bible college. Then up the coast to Sydney where we stayed at a mission guest house and visited with local missionaries. After speaking in a church in Brisbane, our hosts took us to a nature preserve. We enjoyed observing the koala bears and brilliant birds of the parrot family.

On to New Zealand we proceeded. We rented a car in Auckland and visited missionary friends there. In Feilding, we spent a glorious weekend with the Church of Christ. One of the active members was a young man who had stayed in our home in Pua before he became a Christian. We visited friends in Wellington and enjoyed many scenic wonders of North Island. In many ways our visit to New Zealand took on a comical tone due to linguistic differences in American English and the New Zealand dialect.

As we did on every furlough trip, we asked our children what site they would most like to visit on their way to the United States. They all wanted to see the Inca Ruins of Machu Picchu in Peru.

Our flight on New Zealand Airways toward Lima developed engine trouble and made an unscheduled stop in Tahiti. What a beautiful island.

We saw a singing and dancing competition involving Tahiti and surrounding islands. The choirs sang in haunting melodies and rich harmony. Singers and dancers wore bright native costumes with wreaths of real flowers. The program was just a short walk from our hotel.

The airline took care of our hotel charges, but the food was out-of-range for our budget. We were offered a rattle-trap car with bald tires for a modest fee. We found a back-alley noodle shop where we could afford to eat.

After a night in the hotel, we drove to view the black sand beaches on the island's east side. Then south to the Gauguin museum to view paintings of the famous French artist who exiled himself to Tahiti. When it was time to leave for the airport, the old buggy rattled, wheezed, and died.

We were in a state of panic, but the charming assistant curator calmed our fears. "I will take you to the airport. Don't worry about the rental car. I know the owner and will have him pick it up."

She took us to the airport and then helped us unload our luggage, then graciously refused our payment offer and wished us Godspeed.

We arrived in Lima before dawn. Peru's capital is a gloomy place and the residents seldom see sunlight. The next morning we took a half-mile walk to the travel agency to cancel our trip to Machu Picchu. Tahiti had nearly exhausted our travel funds.

The gracious travel agent said, "Your children have traveled halfway around the world. They should not have to miss Machu Picchu." She proceeded to make our round-trip plane tickets to Cuzco, two nights at the hotel there, and round-trip train tickets to the ruins of Machu Picchu.

"How can we ever thank you?" I asked. "Just pass it on when you can," she said with a smile. Why should we continue to be surprised at unexpected provision?

The transition from sea-level Lima to the Andean mountain heights of Cuzco caused Dorothy and the girls to experience the miseries of altitude sickness. A solicitous steward of the hotel brewed some coca leaf tea.

While the girls recovered at the hotel, Geoffrey and I explored the magnificent stone structures of the ancient Incas and the arts and handicrafts of their modern descendants. It was a preparation for the awesome architecture of Machu Picchu which we would explore the next day.

The train ride through the Andean slopes took four hours. What a glorious time we had clambering through the terraces and structures of these marvelous ruins.

From Lima we proceeded through Mexico City to Dallas and finally St. Louis. Dorothy's brother, Sam Dyson, met us at the airport there. He drove us to their hometown of Chandlerville and a reunion with Grandma Dyson and family. We were finally back in the beloved country that could never again be fully our home.

Study Questions

1. Garland described the journey back to the United States with word pictures of the beauty the family enjoyed. What a refreshing time God provided for the family! Were you surprised when their rental car episode turned out just fine? Or when the travel agent provided a way to see the ruins of Machu Picchu? Would either of these meet your description of a miracle?

2. Read Psalm 117:2 and Psalm 63:3. What should be our response when we soak in the refreshment of God's goodness and lovingkindness?

3. Read Matthew 5:7. When you give of yourself to serve God, what happens?

Chapter 20

Reentry into America

Upon our return from Thailand I received eight offers of medical positions. A physician shortage had accompanied the end of the Vietnam War. Each offer had its own attractions, especially those with a missionary flavor including a clinic serving the impoverished in Appalachia and an Indian reservation in Montana. I had not applied for any of the positions.

My parents had retired to Lincoln, Nebraska, my mother's hometown. They lived in a cottage across the street from the Douglas Street Church of Christ where my sister Marguerite served with her husband Archie Fairbrother.

How could we purchase a home and an automobile without credit history? How could I catch up on continuing medical education while needing to work full time? We had no experience with owning a credit card or borrowing money.

Anxiety stretched faith to its limits. Reassurance came from unexpected sources. "Chance encounters" began to look like divine appointments. The upshot was a position offer from the University of Nebraska Health Center. Park School offered the special education and physical therapy that Grace Eileen needed. We found all our immediate needs met in Lincoln, Nebraska.

We immediately plunged into efforts to begin a campus ministry. Initially called College-Career Christian Fellowship. I also started a sub-group called Medical Careers Christian Fellowship. Students preparing for careers in medicine, dentistry, nursing, pharmacy, and other health-related fields met monthly. Christian professionals from these fields came and lectured on opportunities for serving Christ through these professions.

We started a Saturday Night Open House in our home as an alternative to the campus party scene. The program consisted of conversation and refreshments with no formal Bible studies. The ministry of hospitality led to a number of decisions to follow Christ. Many of the participants are now serving Christ in various parts of the world.

Many students asked to be mentored. Since this could not be done during working hours, we met for brown bag lunches either in the football stadium or the Coliseum during the noon hour.

The University asked me to teach classes in health sciences. In addition, the fraternities and sororities invited me to give in-house lectures on various health topics.

In 1977, the University appointed me as Medical Director with the rank of Dean. The monthly Deans and Directors meeting gave an insight into the inner workings of university administration. At the beginning of my term, I set five goals for the University Health Services. We achieved all of these goals by 1981, so I returned to full-time patient care and teaching. I also joined part-time the Lincoln Family Medical Group, a partnership of Christian physicians with offices in Lincoln and Ashland.

Working mainly with college students, I had missed delivering babies and assisting surgery. Guiding young couples through pregnancy and delivery has its own special joys, especially when one can pray with the young parents.

Heavy involvement with the church, campus ministry, and medical practice led to deep heartache. I realized it would not be possible to fulfill my Nebraska responsibilities and still remain in active contact with our beloved Thailand. My shoulders were not broad enough to carry two far-flung ministries.

The believers in Thailand were deeply grieved that I was not maintaining correspondence with them. Letters from Thailand brought heart-rending questions. "How have we offended you so deeply that you do not write to us anymore? Do you still remember to pray for us? Our struggles would be easier if you encouraged us."

Dorothy kept busy with Laubach Literacy and Teaching English as a Second Language to the refugees who flooded in. The disabilities of my parents' old age required more and more care and time. Dorothy handled doctor visits, banking, and grocery shopping for them, especially after my father could no longer drive.

When Grace Eileen left home to marry to marry Rodney Meester, Sr., Dorothy had more free time for her other duties. Father went to his eternal reward just short of his 94th birthday. Mother lived to be 96 years old. After their departure, Dorothy spent several years homeschooling three grandchildren. Lisa Castillo came to live with us at age sixteen and became another beloved daughter.

After twenty exciting years, I retired from the University at age 65 in 1995. The next six years would be spent full time with Lincoln Family Medical Group. Due to higher insurance premiums and greater risks I had stopped delivering babies in 1989.

Study Questions

1. "Anxiety stretches faith to its limits" with all the immediate needs for housing, education, and transportation. Read Psalm 84:11, Matthew 6:31-32 and Philippians 4:19. How many of the Bare family's need were met?

2. With the hospitality and refreshments of the Saturday Night Open Houses came a number of decisions to follow Christ. How could that happen with no formal Bible studies going on?

3. Read 2 Corinthians 3:2-3. Does your life – and your heart – reflect the love of Christ? It's more about who you are than what you say. Living a life that reflects the heart of Jesus is what will draw people to Him. Our goal should be to pursue Jesus' transformation and love so completely that we reflect His heart to the world.

4. Do you agree with this statement: "We can get the gospel message to a broken world by living and loving like Jesus."

Epilogue

Return Visit to Thailand

In late 1997 the opportunity arose for Dorothy and me to return to Thailand briefly. We experienced a twenty-three year absence after being on the field for twenty-three years. How exciting it would be to return to the scene of our labors and reunite with the national believers and fellow missionaries.

Among the encouragers urging us to make the trip were Ned and Linda Stringham. Linda was a "charter member" of the campus ministry and a talented encourager. Her witty writing brightened the stress-filled moments of campus life for many students.

Ned, a graduate of Carnegie-Mellon University, came to the Saturday Night Open House his first night in Lincoln, Nebraska. Ned and Linda met through the campus ministry and I was privileged to participate in their wedding. Ned earned a Ph.D. in psychology and counseling and was a charter member of Lincoln Counseling and Enrichment Associates, partnering with Lincoln Family Group to treat the whole person.

The trip to Thailand was eventful. From Lincoln we connected to a jumbo jet in Minneapolis. A strong headwind forced an unscheduled refueling stop at Anchorage. The extra hours in the air led to a missed connection in Osaka and non-functioning restrooms on the plane. (Don't try to imagine the smell.)

Complicating the trip, a Filipino lady passenger had a significant cardiac event just an hour out of Osaka. The call came over the loudspeaker, "Is there a doctor on the plane? Urgent help is needed at the front of the cabin!"

Hesitating a moment to see if anyone else responded, I pulled my stethoscope out of my briefcase and rushed forward. The flight attendant had placed the distressed patient on oxygen. Grabbing the microphone, I asked if any passengers had nitroglycerin. Immediately several bottles were thrust forward. I gave her the appropriate dose. I asked the plane crew to radio Osaka for an ambulance to be at the plane entrance when we disembarked. The flight attendants needed to keep all passengers on board until the ambulance had loaded and departed.

Months later I received a letter from the airline thanking me for my intervention and giving me a voucher for a future flight. Enclosed was a thank-you note from the patient's husband informing me that his wife had made a good recovery.

The airline accommodated us in a hotel in Osaka since we had missed our Miyazaki connection. We called Al and Rhonda Juve, missionaries in Miyazaki telling them we would arrive the following morning. Al had been a student at the University of Nebraska when I first met him. He was in the drug world four years and had an interest in Tibet. It fascinated him that I had lived in Tibet, and he sought opportunities to question me. Sometime after he started coming to the Saturday Night Open House, he committed his life to Christ.

Al's spiritual transformation reversed the damage done by drugs. He transferred to Nebraska Christian College (NCC) where he made the dean's list for scholastic achievement every semester. At NCC he met and married Rhonda Schwarz, a highly capable and accomplished young woman, the valedictorian of her class.

After our night in Osaka, we flew over the beautiful islands to Kyushu the sub-tropical southern-most island. Al and Rhonda met us at the Miyazaki airport. We had a scenic tour of the island and enjoyed the hospitality of their home. Al insisted that I take the time to tell his precocious daughters, Sarah and Laura, stories of my childhood in Tibet. (At this writing Al and Rhonda Juve have completed thirty years as missionaries to Japan.)

Back to Thailand

As our plane descended into the Bangkok airport, we felt high anticipation mingled with dread. We had been informed that Bangkok traffic had increased to the point that it often took four hours to cover the thirty miles into the city. The stifling humidity blasted us as we stepped off the plane. Our arrival coincided with a national holiday, the King's Birthday, so traffic was greatly diminished. I had retained enough of the language to bargain our taxi fare down to a reasonable amount. To our delight, the trip into the city took less than an hour.

Joy Boese, who had been one of the nurses at the Maranatha Clinic twenty-seven years earlier, had arranged for our stay at the CMA Guest House. In our guest room she provided a welcoming basket of the fruit we had missed. These included melt-in-your-mouth *mangosteens,* brown-sugary *lamuts,* and spiky *rambutans* with their grape-like interiors.

Dick and Beulah Johnston were our cordial hosts at the Guest House. We had known them when they were young missionaries working with the Cambodian-speaking peoples of Northeast Thailand. Beulah was the sister of Bill Smalley, the American Bible Society representative who had been our advisor in the Bible translation days.

Our first Sunday back in Thailand, Dick took us out to the Asia Institute of Technology to preach at the Sunday morning services to students from all the nations of Southeast Asia. It was delightful to join with engineering students from Thailand, Indonesia, Malaysia, India, the Philippines, and Korea in singing the praises of our God.

Joy was our guide through the vastly changed streets of Bangkok. Doctors from my Chiang Mai Medical School class hosted us at a sumptuous banquet. We marveled at the skyscrapers that now dominated the Bangkok skyline.

Reunion with Missionaries

In Chiang Mai we stayed in the home of David and Deloris Filbeck. Since starting their mission work in Pua, they had made impressive strides in language reduction, translations, and evangelism with the Lua tribe. Now they were starting a Bible training school in Chiang Mai with the help of their grown children.

At the Filbeck home, Deloris arranged a reception for missionaries we had known. What a joy to refresh ourselves in the company of those who had touched our lives. These included Dr. Edwin McDaniel, who had encouraged me to begin my pre-medical studies at Wheaton College, Janet Greenleaf former nurse at Maranatha, and members of the Morse family. We also got to visit with Daniel and Bev Kalnin and learn about their

"Barefoot Doctors" program in Burma. Virgilio and Esther de los Santos introduced us to their new work in Chiang Mai. Their children had grown into active participants in the work.

How convenient to be able to travel all-weather roads where we once walked mountain trails. We traveled by bus to Chiangkham to spend a few days with Dorothy Uhlig. The scene of our first two years in Thailand had become thoroughly modern. Television, computers, and cell phones were commonplace. Automobiles crowded paved streets.

Our first Sunday morning we drove up to a Hmong village. Being among believers in that tribe brought great joy.

During the week I sat in on Dorothy Uhlig's clinic. In the early days of the clinic, patient problems concerned nutritional disease, malaria, and worms. Now, she was dealing with AIDS and narcotic abuse.

In 1951, our first Sunday services were at the leprosy village of Sope Waan. We went by bicycle through the paddy fields. The church met in a bamboo hut under a grass roof.

Now, forty-six years later we took a bus out to a cement worship center in the village. They had built a concrete chapel with a large courtyard. It was no longer a leprosy village, but many of the members were grandchildren of the original leprosy patients. They conducted the services in the courtyard, having outgrown the building.

Back in Chiang Mai we attended English-language services at the International Church in the evening. We met and renewed acquaintance with many more missionaries.

EPILOGUE

The Medical Work

Doctors in the Chiang Mai Hospital, who had been my classmates in medical school, entertained us with a banquet. The following day I went back to the medical school to visit my old professors while Dorothy toured the city with Deloris Filbeck.

The physiology professor invited me to lunch at his home. His daughter had attended Abilene Christian College and was married to a Church of Christ missionary.

Another visit was to Dr. Charn, who had been one of my instructors in Internal Medicine. Famous for his strictness, the students were afraid of him. I found that the years had not mellowed him. He introduced me to his class, "This is Dr. Garland Bare, the only American to graduate from Chiang Mai Medical College. He was not very bright but did manage to graduate."

What a surprise to return to Pua. All-weather highways made it a relatively quick drive from Chiang Mai. No longer was Pua a village of oxcart trails and thatch-roofed huts. Modern concrete buildings gleamed along paved streets. My little, ten-bed hospital had been replaced by a shining three-story building with multiple departments. The Crown Prince of Thailand had endowed the hospital.

A few members of the original hospital staff introduced the new staff and gave a tour of the various departments. The reality exceeded my wildest dreams. Near the hospital was a small but modern airport.

The doctors treated us to a luncheon and honored me as "the Grandfather of the Pua Hospital." Three of the young people who were in the hostel in the 1970s served in the medical profession: Sawang as an Emergency Room Technologist, Manop as a Radiology Tech in a district hospital, and Jarunee as a nurse.

The Hostel

Gratitude to God. Joy in their growth. Pride in their achievements. These emotions flooded our hearts as we returned to the scene of our involvement with tribal children. Among the first students, Panya shone for his academic achievements and faithful service. At the time of our visit, he taught agriculture in the Wang Pa High School. He also maintained a hostel for tribal youngsters and preached in Hmong villages.

Suljin worked in the Paklang church. He had also made trips to the United States to preach to Hmong refugees in Minnesota and Wisconsin.

Jaratsi had married Peter Sutjaibun of the Rawang tribe. They attended Cincinnati Bible Seminary where she adopted the name Ruth Sutjaibun. She and Peter returned to Thailand as teachers.

Pak Dee had attended Bible school and evangelized the Hmong in the Chiang Mai region. We visited in his home and were delighted to meet his mother, Xaiv Suav's widow.

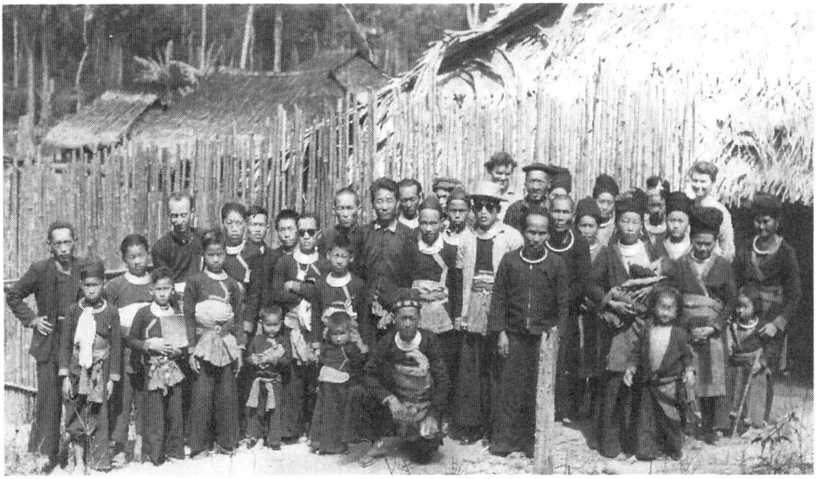

Hmong believers outside grass and bamboo chapel

As mentioned earlier, Sawang, Manop, and Jarunee were involved in medical work and faithful to the Lord. Juralee and her husband were working with the United Nations in Kosovo, but visited Paklang while we were there.

The fact that some who once testified to strong faith had fallen away tempered our joy. We also grieved for those who had shown so much promise but failed to follow the Lord.

The strong encouragement of Imogene Williams and Hmong believers has kept the hostel going. Since Imogene's return to the States, a Hmong alumna has maintained it as a girl's hostel.

Agriculture

Opium was the main cash crop of the highland tribes. With belief in Christ, the tribespeople came to the conviction that growing and marketing narcotics violated Christian conduct. In the early years, we had converted the hillside behind our home into an experimental plot for fruit and nut trees and tea and coffee bushes.

How delighted we were on our return to find the opium fields all gone and the hillsides covered with orchards. Trees in orderly rows produced crops of lychees, longans, and peaches. They marketed their produce as far away as Bangkok. In exploring the orchards, Dorothy and I, for the first time, were able to travel on paved roads to high mountain villages and the Bau Valley salt wells.

Final Adventure

Back in Chiang Mai, I had the privilege of meeting and traveling with Aaron, an evangelist from the Lahu tribe. After graduating from Lincoln Christian College, he had returned to preach and plant churches among the Lahu. Fluency in Thai and English allowed him to become business manager for some of the missionaries.

In early January 1998, Aaron invited me to preach in a new Lahu congregation on the Burma border. The day before our proposed trip, Aaron called to say that the village headman had decreed that we and our vehicle would be stoned if we preached in the village.

"Shall we go?" asked Aaron.

"I never heard of the apostle Paul avoiding a stoning party," I replied.

Dorothy remained in Chiang Mai to attend services with the Filbecks. Aaron and I started at dawn. As our vehicle climbed into the village, I admit to glancing nervously left and right for stone flingers.

All was quiet as we pulled up to the little bamboo chapel. Half of the congregation stayed away from the service because of the headmaster's threats. I preached in Northern Thai and Aaron interpreted into Lahu.

Partway through the service there was a nervous stir as the assistant headman walked into the chapel. He stood in the back while Aaron and I continued to preach.

After the service, he earnestly began to question Aaron. He asked permission to ride in our vehicle to the next village so that he could continue his questions.

In 1999, Aaron called me from Lincoln Christian College where he was working on his master's degree. The headman and assistant headman had been baptized, and the church was thriving.

⌖ ⌖ ⌖

The return visit had helped us catch up on our friends of the past. JunTa, the Sorcerer, had been a faithful clinic evangelist as long as his health permitted. Saeng Pua, the Outlaw, Uncle Tip, the seeker, and Grandfather Gaao had all completed their pilgrimage, faithful to the end. Tswv Sab, the Bear Feeder, was in the final stages of cancer, but still clinging to the faith. Panya continued his faithful service.

How blessed we were to see God rewarding our labors and continuing to bless his followers in Thailand.

"Now to him who is able to do far more abundantly than all we ask or think, according to the power at work within us, to him be glory in the church and in Christ Jesus through all generations, forever and ever."

- Ephesians 3: 20-21